The Silent Struggles:
UNDERSTANDING WOMEN'S MENTAL HEALTH

Break The Stigma, Prioritize Self-Care, Reach Out

For The Support Thereby

Empowering Mental Health.

DR. DINESH KANFADE

ACKNOWLEDGEMENTS

I wish to express my gratitude to various sources, knowingly or unknowingly has contributed for empowering my knowledge, empowering women's health and helping me to write this book.

I would like to thank my mentors and teachers who had been a torch bearer for me for writing this book.

I am extremely thankful to **Adv. (Dr.) Ashok Yende**, Ex-Professor & HOD, Department of Law, Mumbai University for taking time from his busy schedule to write **"FOREWORD"** for my book.

I am also extremely thankful to **Dr. Nalini Kurvey**, Sr. Obstetrician & Gynecologist for taking time from her busy schedule to write **"FOREWORD"** for my book.

I also express my sincere gratitude to my family members especially my wife Nita, son Akshay and friends who have always been supportive and motivated me in my initiatives in writing series of books on **"Women's Health"**, this book being sixth in the series.

DEDICATION

Dedicated to my better half Nita,
son Akshay, daughter-in-law Priya
and little sweet Avni.

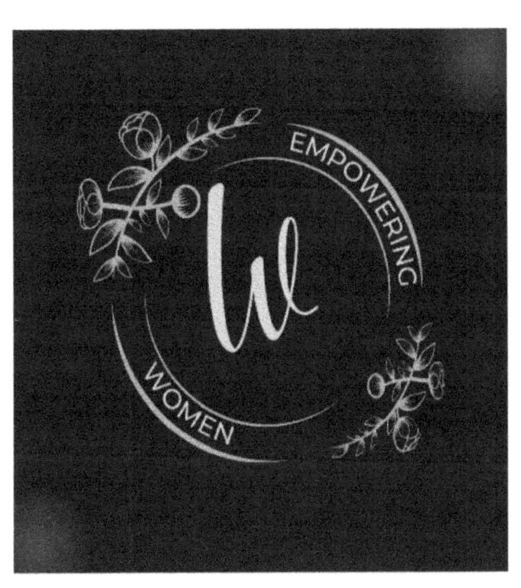

EMPOWERING
WOMEN
W

*"Women are more than twice as likely as men
to get an anxiety disorder in their lifetime.
In addition, women may face challenges with
their hormones, reproductive mental health
and being victims of abuse."*

"Each year 1 in 5 women in the United States

has a mental health problem such as depression,

post-traumatic stress disorder (PTSD),

or an eating disorder."

And there are many other challenges

women can face with their mental health

and emotional wellness."

-American Psychiatric Association

"Our greatest glory is not in never falling,

But rising in every time we fall."

-Confucius

FOREWORD:

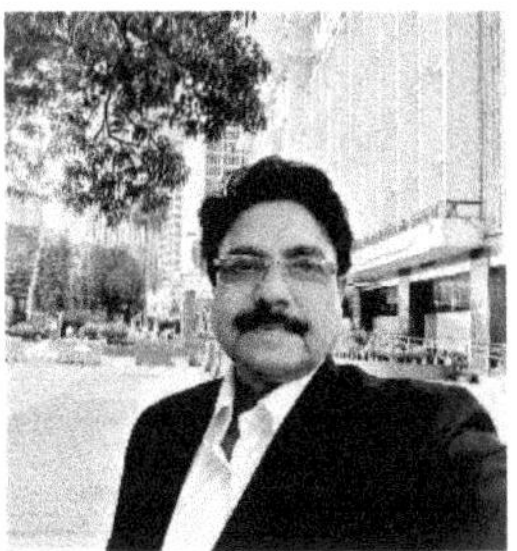

In an era where the mental health conversation is growing, the struggles faced by women often remain muted, misunderstood, and marginalized. The book **"The Silent Struggles: Understanding Women's Mental Health"** sheds light on the critical phases of a woman's life – adolescence, reproductive years, and menopause – and how each phase brings unique challenges to her mental well-being. In this book, the author delves deep into issues such as child marriages, societal pressures, and the often-overlooked mental scars left by heinous acts like sexual and physical assault.

The recurrence of heinous acts such as the recent physical and sexual assault of a junior doctor at R. G. Kar Medical College Kolkata (August 2024), the infamous Nirbhaya case (2012), and many others reveal several ground realities. These incidents highlight the persistent shortcomings, and complexities of our justice delivery system, and the failure of police administration where delayed justice, inadequate protection for victims, and lack of stringent punishment for perpetrators, contribute to the recurrence of such crimes. Delayed justice can exacerbate the trauma and suffering of the victim. The uncertainty and prolonged wait for a decision can have severe psychological and emotional impacts. I appreciate the role of the Supreme Court, and High Courts in taking Suo motu cognizance of some such brutal rape cases, addressing the issues, and leading to law, and policy changes. The criminalization of politics and politicization of the police system lead to delay in filing first information reports (FIR), and influence the crime investigation, allowing criminals to go unpunished, raising concerns of a public safety threat by criminals remaining free. Through detailed exploration, the book brings much-needed awareness to the long-lasting effects of these violent encounters on the victim's mental health if she survives. As a society, we can better address and support their recovery in collaboration with government/non-government, or civil society organisations. This book is not just an exploration but a call to action - a reminder that understanding these silent struggles is the first step towards empowering the women who face them. This book identifies and analyses some of the problems women victims are facing, and tries to suggest remedial measures.

Dr. Dinesh Kanfade, a visionary Obstetrician & Gynaecologist with more than 35 years of experience offers a unique perspective on understanding women's mental health, which can benefit anyone interested in improving their understanding of this subject. The author's writing style is engaging, the book is well-structured, clearly and concisely explaining the subject matter. In my opinion, it's an excellent choice for healthcare professionals, educators, and anyone seeking to truly understand the complexities of women's mental health and gain a deeper understanding of the topic covered in the book.

ADV. (DR.) ASHOK YENDE

B.Sc. LLB, LLM, Ph.D. (M.U.); Ph.D. (Texas, USA), D.Lit.

Founder & CEO, Yende Legal Associates
Mediator, Bombay High Court & Mah. State Consumer Commission
Ombudsperson (Lokpal), National Law University, Mumbai
Professor & Former Head, Department of Law, University of Mumbai.

FOREWORD:

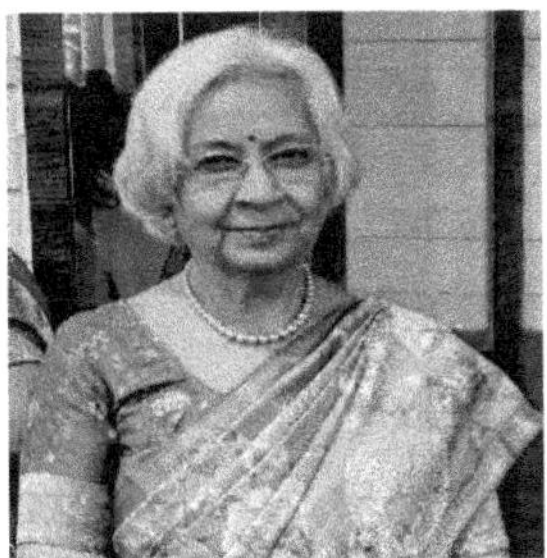

It gives me great pleasure to present the book, **"The Silent Struggles: Understanding Women's Mental Health"**, written by Dr. Dinesh Kanfade.

The book, **"The Silent Struggles: Understanding Women's Mental Health"**, is an essential read for healthcare providers, caregivers and women of all ages. The author has meticulously explored the mental health challenges that women face during adolescence, child marriages, reproductive years, menopause, and during physical / sexual violence; shedding light on issues that are often misunderstood or overlooked.

As a healthcare professional, I seek the critical need for resources that address the unique health experiences of women. This book not only provides valuable knowledge but also encourages a compassionate approach to care. It reminds us that each stage of women's life brings distinct mental health considerations that deserve attention and understanding. **"The Silent Struggles: Understanding Women's Mental Health"**, offers a comprehensive framework that can guide practitioners in delivering more empathetic and effective care.

For every woman, whether you are young adolescent navigating the tumultuous journey of self-discovery, a mother balancing the demands of life and family, a woman entering menopause and facing new challenges, or a woman facing challenges due to physical/sexual violence; this book is a must read. It empowers women with the knowledge to advocate for their mental well-being. I highly recommend this book as an invaluable resource for anyone committed to improving women's mental health across all stages of life.

DR. NALINI KURVEY

MD, DGO.

Sr. Obstetrician & Gynaecologist

Vice-President, Association of Medical Women in India (AMWI)

Ex-President, Nagpur Obstetric & Gynaecological Society

Director, Kurvey Maternity & Nursing Home, Nagpur.

PREFACE:

In recent years, the importance of women's health has gained much needed attention, yet mental health remains an area often overlooked or misunderstood. Throughout history, women's voices have been marginalized, their experiences often dismissed or misunderstood. This book, **"The Silent Struggles: Understanding Women's Mental Health"**, is an attempt to bridge this gap, providing a comprehensive exploration of the mental health challenges faced by women at different stages of life.

Additionally, domestic and work-place violence has long been a major concern for women globally, including in India.

The journey begins with an introductory chapter that underscores the critical importance of women's health as a foundation for societal well-being. Following this, the focus shifts to adolescent girls, examining the mental health challenges they face, including the impact of child marriages – a practice still prevalent in many parts of the world.

The discussion moves to women of reproductive age, where the intricacies of mental health are closely tied to the demands of parenthood. Here, the book delves into how a parental mental health significantly affect child development, underscoring the intergenerational impact of mental wellness.

Next chapter addresses the often-neglected phase of menopause, exploring the mental health issues that arises as women transition through this significant phase of life.

Additionally, the challenges faced by girls/women due to physical/sexual violence such as recent incidence of sexual and physical assault on junior doctor of R. G. Medical College Kolkata (August 2024) and the impact of these incidents on mental health cannot be ignored.

This book is intended to serve as a resource for healthcare professionals, educators, women of all ages and anyone interested in understanding the complex landscape of women's mental health, providing both knowledge and empathy in equal measure.

DR. DINESH KANFADE

MBBS. DGO. DFP. FICMCH. CIMP.

Sr. Obstetrician & Gynecologist.

Table of Content:

CHAPTER I: INTRODUCTION

"Taking care for your mental health is an act of self-love.

But there is no shame in seeking help

for your mental health issues."

(A) Definition of Mental Health

Mental illness is a health issue. It can affect your thoughts, mood or behavior. It can impact the way you perceive the world around you.

Mental health encompasses emotional, psychological and social wellbeing influencing cognition, perception and behavior.

Mental illness can last for a short time or for your whole life. Some mild health illness last only for a few weeks. But some severe illnesses can be life-long and can cause severe disability.

According to WHO (World Health Organization):

Mental health is defined as "A state of wellbeing in which the individual realizes his or her abilities, can cope with the normal stresses of life, can work productively and fruitfully and can contribute to his or her community."

In other words, mental health determines how an individual handles stress, interpersonal relationships and decision-making with normal stresses of life.

From the perspectives of positive psychology and holism, mental health may include an individual's ability to enjoy life and to create a balance between life activities and efforts to achieve psychological resilience.

Mental health is a basic human right.

It is crucial for individual, family, community

and socio-economic development.

Some Early Signs in Relation to Mental Health include:

- Unusual or illogical thoughts
- Lack of Energy
- Sleep disturbances
- Poor concentration and memory
- Unreasonable anger and irritability
- Thinking of harming oneself or others
- Lack of motivation
- Increased or low appetite
- Feelings that life is not worth living or suicidal thoughts
- Self- Isolation

Determinants of Mental Health:

Here are some key determinants of mental health.

- **Biological Factors:**
  Genetics, brain chemistry and hormonal imbalances can influence mental health conditions.

- **Psychological Factors:**
  Personality traits, coping mechanisms, cognitive patterns and early life experiences play a significant role.

- **Social Factors:**
  Relationships, social support networks, family dynamics and community connections impact mental wellbeing.

- **Environmental Factors:**
  Stressors such as trauma, abuse, poverty, discrimination and access to resources all affect mental health.

- **Lifestyle Factors:**
  Exercise, diet, substance abuse, sleep patterns and overall self-care practices contribute to mental health.

- **Cultural Factors:**
  Cultural benefits, values, norms and attitudes towards mental health and seeking help shape individual's experiences.

- **Economic Factors:**
  Socioeconomic status, employment opportunities and financial stability can impact mental health outcomes.

- **Access to Healthcare:**
  Availability and affordability of mental health services, as well as stigma surrounding seeking help, influence access to care.

(B) Magnitude of the Problem:

Mental Health Issue Globally:

According to **World Health Organization (WHO),** 970 million people worldwide were living with some form of a mental disorder in 2019, which is every 1 in 8 people. The most common mental disorders are anxiety and depression.

Here are some other mental health statistics:

- 1 in every 4 people will be affected by a mental illness at some point in their lives.

- 350 million people worldwide suffer from depression.

- 14.3% of deaths worldwide, or approximately 8 million deaths each year, are attributed to mental illness.

- People with several mental health conditions die 10 – 20 years earlier than the general population.

- Having a mental health condition, increases the risk of suicidal tendencies and experiencing human rights violations.

- Almost 9 out of 10 people with a mental condition experience stigma and discrimination, which negatively affect their lives.

- A study published in September 2022 estimates that the global burden of mental illness in 2019 was 418 million disability-adjusted life years

(DALYs), which is more than three-fold increase from various estimates. The economic value associated with this burden is estimated at about USD 5 trillion.

Mental Health Issues in India:

- According to a 2016 National Health Survey, 5.1% of Indians have common mental disorders, such as anxiety and depressive disorders.

- However, estimates suggest that nearly 15% of the Indian population has some form of mental health issue. This figure encompasses many disorders including anxiety disorders, depression, bipolar disorders, schizophrenia, substance use disorders and neurodevelopmental disorders.

- **According to 2018 WHO report**, India is the 6th most depressed country in the world. WHO also reports India, China and United States are the most affected countries by anxiety, schizophrenia and bipolar disorders.

- According to a **2023 Mckinsey Health Institute Survey**, India ranks second in the world for fostering mental wellbeing at workplaces.

- India is considered the world's suicide capital, with 2.6 lakh cases of suicide in a year.

Rank of India in Mental Health:

According to 2024 World Happiness Report, India ranks 126th out of 143 countries for happiness levels. The reports consider factors such as social support, income, health, freedom, generosity and the absence of corruption.

(C) Comparison of Mental Health Issues in Women and Men:

- Globally, mental health issues disproportionately affect women. According to **WHO**, depression is more common in women than men, with an estimated 4.4% of women experienced depression compared to 3.6% of men.

- Anxiety disorders also affect women more frequently, with women being approximately twice more likely to experience anxiety disorders compared to men.

- Women are also more likely to experience trauma-related mental health conditions, such as PTSD (posttraumatic stress disorder), due to factors such as gender-based violence and sexual assault.

- Eating disorders, including anorexia nervosa and bulimia, predominantly affect women, often stemming from societal pressures related to body image and beauty standards.

- Women may engage in self-harm behaviors as a coping mechanism for distress, and suicidal rates among young girls are rising globally.

- In India, the prevalence of mental illness among women is significant as per the **Lancet Psychiatry Journal Report**. About 14.7% of Indian women suffer from mental illness, with depression being the most common disorder.

- **The National Health Survey of India conducted in 2016** found that the prevalence of common mental disorders (CMD) among women was 7.5%, compared to 4.6% among men.

- Women in India face unique challenges such as gender-based discrimination, societal expectations and limited access to mental health services, which contribute to higher prevalence of mental health issues.

- Despite the higher incidence of mental illnesses in women, there are disparities in diagnosis and treatment. Women may be less likely to seek help due to stigma, financial constraints or lack of awareness about available resources.

- Gender biases in the healthcare system can also result in underdiagnoses or misdiagnosis of mental health conditions in women, leading to inadequate treatment.

- Socioeconomic factors such as poverty, education level and access to healthcare significantly influence women's mental health outcomes. Women with marginalized communities or lower socioeconomic backgrounds may face greater barriers to accessing mental health services.

(D) How Women's Mental Health Differ from that of Men's and what are the Unique Challenges?

- **Hormonal Variations:**
  Women experience hormonal fluctuations throughout their menstrual cycles, pregnancy, childbirth and menopause, which can affect mood regulation and mental health differently than men.

- **Social Expectations and Roles:**
  Societal norms and expectations regarding gender roles may place pressure on women, influencing their mental health. For example, women may face more expectations, related to caregiving and managing household responsibilities.

- **Psychological Factors:**
  Women may be more prone to certain psychological disorders such as depression and anxiety, which can be influenced by factors such as hormonal changes, societal pressures and coping mechanisms.

- **Trauma and Violence:**
  Women are more likely to experience gender-based violence, sexual assault and domestic abuse, which can have significant impact on their mental health as compared to men.

- **Body Image and Self-Esteem:**
  Societal pressure related to appearance and body image can disproportionately affect women than men, leading to issues such as eating disorders and low self-esteem, which can impact mental health.

- **Healthcare Access and Treatment:**
Women may face barriers in accessing mental healthcare, including stigma, financial constraints and lack of awareness about resources. Additionally, women's symptom may be overlooked or underdiagnosed due to gender biases in the healthcare system.

- **Reproductive Health:**
Issues related to reproductive health, such as infertility, pregnancy related complications and postpartum depression, can significantly impact women's mental wellbeing.

- **Social Support Network:**
Women may tend to have stronger mental support networks and be more likely to seek help from friends, family or support groups, which can positively influence their mental health outcomes compared to men.

- **Coping Mechanisms:**
Women may adopt different coping categories than men in response to stressors, which can impact their mental health outcomes. For example, women may be more likely to seek social support or engage in expressive form of coping, such as talking about their feelings.

- **Intersectionality:**
Women's mental health experiences are also influenced by intersecting factors such as race, ethnicity, sexual orientation and socioeconomic status, which can compound the challenges they face and affect their access to resources and support.

(E) Importance of Women's Mental Health

By prioritizing women's mental health, individuals including families, communities and societies as a whole can recap numerous benefits, leading to healthier, happier and more prosperous outcomes for everyone.

- **Individual Wellbeing:**
  - **Improved quality of life:**
    Good mental health allows women to enjoy a high quality of life, experiencing greater emotional wellbeing and fulfillment.

  - **Enhanced Coping Skills:**
    Strong mental health equips women with effective coping mechanism to navigate life's challenges and stressors.

  - **Increased Productivity:**
    Better mental health enables women to be more productive in their personal and professional endeavors.

- **Family Dynamics:**
  - **Positive Parenting:**
    Women with good mental health can provide nurturing and supportive environment for their children, providing healthy development and wellbeing.

  - **Stronger Relationships:**
    Good mental health fosters stronger and more fulfilling relationships with partners, children and extended family members.

- o **Effective Communication:**
  Women with good mental health can communicate with more effectively, resolving conflicts and fostering harmony within the family unit.

- **Community Wellbeing:**
  - o **Support Network:**
    Women with good mental health can actively participate in community support networks, providing assistance and solidarity to others facing mental health challenges.

  - o **Advocacy and Awareness:**
    Mentally healthy women can advocate for mental health awareness and resources within their communities, reducing stigma and promoting access to care.

  - o **Civic Engagement:**
    Mentally healthy women are more likely to engage in civic activities and community initiatives, contributing to the societal fabric and wellbeing of their communities.

- **Societal Advancement:**
  - o **Economic Impact:**
    Women with good mental health are better positioned to participate in the workforce, driving economic growth and stability for themselves and society.

  - o **Reduced Healthcare Costs:**
    Prevention and treatment of mental health issues among women can lead to significant cost savings by reducing the burden on

healthcare systems and increasing overall productivity.

- o **Social Cohesion:**
  Supporting women's mental health contributes to greater social cohesion and resilience, fostering a more inclusive and equitable society for all members.

(F) Historical Aspects of Mental Health

Here is historical perspective on how mental health issues among women have been perceived and treated over time.

- **Ancient Times:**
  - o In ancient civilizations, mental health issues were often attributed to supernatural causes or divine punishment.

  - o Women experiencing mental health symptoms might be seen as possessed by evil spirits or cursed, leading to stigmatization and isolation.

- **Medieval and Early Modern Period:**
  - o During the medieval and early modern period, mental health issues among women were often interpreted through the lens of religious beliefs and societal norms.

- o Women who displayed unconventional behavior or expressed dissenting opinions could be labelled as witches and subjected to persecution and torture.

- **19th Century:**
  - o The 19th Century saw the emergence of institutions for the care and treatment for the individuals with mental illnesses including women.

  - o However, these institutions often provided harsh and inhuman conditions, with little focus on therapeutic interventions or uncivilized care.

  - o Women who deviated from expected social norms, such as those who expressed strong emotions or challenged patriarchal authority, were particularly vulnerable to confinement and mistreatment.

- **Early 20th Century:**
  - o The early 20th Century witnessed advancement in the understanding of mental health and also the eugenic movements and forced sterilization laws.

  - o Women deemed "feeble-minded" or "morally deficient" were targeted for sterilization as a means of preventing the transmission of mental illness to future generations.

- **Mid to Late 20th Century:**
  - The mid to late 20th Century saw shifts in attitudes towards mental health, with greater emphasis on deinstitutionalization and community-based care.

  - Women's mental health issues, such as depression and anxiety, gained recognition as legitimate conditions, although stigma persisted.

  - The women's liberation movement brought attention to the intersection of gender and mental health, highlighting the impact of societal expectations and gender inequalities on women's wellbeing.

- **21st Century:**
  - In the 21st Century, there has been increased awareness of gender disparities in the mental health diagnosis, treatment and research.

  - Efforts to destigmatize mental illness and promote gender-sensitive approaches to mental health care have gained momentum.

  - However, women still face barriers to accessing mental health services, including socioeconomic factors, cultural beliefs and systemic biases.

Understanding the historical context of how mental health issues among women have been perceived and treated can provide insight into the current challenges and inform efforts to promote gender equity in mental health care. Mental health illness is treatable and their impact can be reduced. However, mental disorders remain among the top ten leading causes of burden on healthcare system worldwide.

In 2017, mental health disorders were the second leading causes of disease burden in terms of years linked with disability and sixth leading causes of disability-adjusted life-years in the world.

While strides have been made in addressing mental health issues globally and in India, there is still much work to be done to address the specific needs of women. Greater awareness, improved access to mental health services, and addressing social determinants of health are crucial in promoting mental wellbeing among women.

(G) Scope and purpose of writing this book:

My book **"The Silent Struggles: Understanding Women's Mental Health"** serves as a vital resource for women, mental health professionals, general practitioners, policymakers and advocates striving to promote mental wellbeing and gender equality.

- **Understanding the Intersectionality of Gender and Mental Health:**
  My book delves into the unique experiences and challenges faced by women in relation to mental health, exploring how gender intersects with other factors such as race, ethnicity, sexuality and socioeconomic status.

- **Raising Awareness and Reducing Stigma:**
  By shedding light on the prevalence and impact of mental health issues among women, my book helps awareness and reduce stigma surrounding women's mental health struggles, encouraging open dialogue and empathy.

- **Providing Resources and Support:**
  My book serves as a comprehensive resource for women, seeking information, support and guidance on managing their mental health. It offers evidence-based strategies, coping mechanisms and self-care practices tailored to women's unique needs.

- **Addressing Societal and Cultural Influences:**
  My book examines the societal and cultural factors that shape women's health experiences, such as gender roles, body image ideals, reproductive health pressures and gender-based

violence. It offers insights into navigating these influences and fostering resilience.

- **Promoting Advocacy and Policy Change:**
  Through highlighting the disparities in mental healthcare access and gender-sensitive policy recommendations, my book empowers readers to advocate for systemic change and greater equity in mental health services for women.

- **Supporting Caregivers and Allies:**
  My book provides valuable guidance for caregivers, partners, family members and allies of women struggling with mental health issues, offering insights into how to provide effective support, foster understanding and promote healing.

- **Fostering Resilience and Empowerment:**
  Ultimately the purpose of my book is to empower women to prioritize their mental health, seek help when needed and cultivate resilience in the face of adversity. It aims to embrace their strengths, advocate for their wellbeing and thrive holistically.

In chapters to follow, this book delves deeper into various aspects of women's mental health, offering insights, strategies and support to empower women, educators in prioritizing women's wellbeing. Each chapter is designed to provide practical tools, resources and inspiration to help readers navigate their mental health journey with confidence and resilience. By addressing mental health in all stages of women's life, my book can provide comprehensive guidance and support tailored to the unique challenges and needs of women in different stages of life. It emphasizes the importance of proactive mental health care throughout the lifespan, promoting resilience, empowerment and holistic wellbeing for women.

CHAPTER II: MENTAL HEALTH IN ADOLESCENCE & YOUNG ADULTHOOD

"Break the stigma, prioritize self-care,

reach out for the support thereby

empowering mental health."

The word adolescence comes from the Latin word adolescere which means "to grow up" or "to mature". It is an unique transitional phase of development that involves rapid physical, cognitive and psychological growth.

World Health Organization (WHO) defines adolescent as someone between the ages 10 and 19 years.

One in every 6 people are aged between 10 and 19 years. Adolescence is the unique stage in life. Physical, emotional and social changes including exposure to poverty, abuse or violence can make adolescents vulnerable to mental health problems.

Mental health conditions are common in adolescent girls, including anxiety, depression, eating disorders and addictive behaviors.

Protecting adolescents from adversity, promoting socio-emotional learning and psychological wellbeing is crucial for their health and wellbeing. Also ensuring access to mental health care is equally important.

According to the World Health Organization (WHO):

- 3.6% of 10 – 14 years old and 4.6% of 15 – 19 years old experience anxiety disorders.

- 1.1% of 10 – 14 years and 2.8% of 15 – 19 years old experience depression.

- *Adolescent girls are about twice as likely to experience depression as compared to boys.*

The major landmark of puberty for female is **menarche** – the appearance of first menses which usually occurs between the ages 12 and 13 years. The onset of puberty in girls is marked by thelarche – development of breast buds which typically occurs after 8 years of age. Thelarche is followed by adrenarche – appearance of axillary and pubic hairs and finally menarche. We will see here systematically the changes during pubertal development and the challenges the adolescent girls have to face during this phase of life and strategies to tackle it.

Pubertal Physical Changes:

(A) Menarche - The first menstrual period in a life of an adolescent girl.

- **Age at Menarche:** Age at menarche varies significantly among girls and the range of factors contribute to this variation.

Typical Age Range:

✓ Average Age around 12.4 years.

✓ Range generally between 10 and 16 years.

✓ Early menarche before 10 years.

✓ Late menarche after 15 years.

- **Factors influencing the age at menarche:**

✓ **Genetics:**

o Approximately half of the variations in age at menarche are attributed to genetically induced factors.

o Family history of early or late menarche can be an indicator.

✓ **Nutritional Status:**

  o Adequate healthy nutrition is essential for healthy development and can influence the age at menarche.

  o In Undernourished or Malnourished girls, menarche can be delayed.

✓ **Body Mass Index (BMI):**

  o Girls with higher BMI are associated with earlier menarche.

  o This may be due to increased production of estradiol, a female sex hormone in adipose tissue.

✓ **Socio-economic Factors:**

  o Girls with higher socio-economic background tend to experience menarche earlier than those from lower socio-economic background.

  o This may be due to better nutrition and overall better living conditions.

✓ **Other Factors:**

  o Ethnic Factors: Ethnic and racial differences can influence age at menarche.

o   Geographical location and/or climate can also play a role.

o   Chronic illnesses and exposure to certain drugs can affect the timing of menarche.

Early and or late menarche may be a sign of underlying medical condition and should be discussed with and investigated as per the advice of healthcare provider.

Impact of Menstruation on Mental Health:

- **Physical Changes:**
  - Adolescent girls may feel unprepared for the physical changes associated with menstruation.

  - There may be inadequate access to sanitary pads, inappropriate school/WASH facilities.

- **Emotional Impact:**
  Menarche may trigger feelings of confusion, embarrassment, or even shame due to stigma and lack of adequate education.

Premenstrual Syndrome (PMS):

- **Physical Symptoms:**
  Symptoms like bloating, breast tenderness and fatigue can disrupt daily activities and affect quality of life.

- **Emotional Symptoms:**
  Mood swings, irritability and anxiety are common, impacting relationships and mental wellbeing.

Premenstrual Dysphoric Disorder (PMDD):

- **Severe Emotional Symptoms:**
  PMDD involves more severe emotional symptoms such as severe depression, irritability and mood swings, which significantly impair daily functioning and quality of life.

- **Impact on Mental Health:**
  PMDD can exacerbate existing mental health conditions like depression and anxiety, leading to increased distress and reduced coping abilities.

Dysmenorrhea (Menstrual Cramps):

- **Pain and Discomfort:**
  Dysmenorrhea involves severe menstrual cramps that can interfere with daily activities, causing absenteeism from schools and work places.

- **Psychological Impact:**
  Chronic pain can lead to feelings of frustration, helplessness and even depression, affecting overall mental wellbeing.

Menorrhagia (Heavy Menstrual Bleeding):

- **Physical Consequences:**
  Excessive bleeding can lead to anemia, fatigue and physical discomfort, affecting day-to-day activities.

- **Emotional Strain:**
  Coping with heavy bleeding and its consequences may lead to anxiety, stress and feelings of inadequacy or embarrassment.

Strategies to Tackle Challenges:

- **Comprehensive Education:**
  - Provide education about menstruation and menstrual health in schools and communities to empower girls with knowledge and reduce stigma.

  - Offer age-appropriate information about the menstrual cycle, hygiene practices and available resources for managing menstrual health.

- **Access to Healthcare:**
  - If a girl hasn't had her periods by the age 13 and hasn't developed secondary sexual characters (such as development of breast buds, axillary and pubic hairs), it is recommended to see a healthcare provider especially a qualified gynaecologist to rule out any underlying medical condition.

  - If a girl hasn't had her periods by the age 13, but has well developed secondary sexual characters and is having monthly cyclical pain in abdomen and is having lumpish feel in lower abdomen or pelvic region, it is recommended to visit healthcare provider. It could be a case of cryptomenorrhea (hidden menstruation due to imperforate hymen) which requires treatment.

  - If the girl hasn't had her periods by the age 15 with developed secondary sexual characters but is suffering from chronic health conditions, it is better to visit healthcare provider for further evaluation.

- ✓ Chronic health conditions such as autoimmune disease like celiac disease, diabetes can delay menarche.

- ✓ Conditions like hypothyroidism and hyperthyroidism can affect hormonal levels, potentially delaying menarche.

- ✓ Eating disorders like anorexia nervosa can affect hormonal levels, further delaying menarche.

- o If a girl hasn't had her periods by the age 15, has well developed secondary sexual characters, no chronic health condition or no other complaints; then her family history needs to be taken into consideration. If a mother or sister started menstruating later than average, it might be normal for the girl to follow a similar pattern.

- o Ensure access to healthcare services for menstrual health concerns, including regular check-ups, screening and treatment options for conditions like PMDD, dysmenorrhea and menorrhagia.

- o Encourage open communication with healthcare providers to address concerns and seek appropriate management strategies.

Delayed menarche can cause anxiety and emotional distress for the girl and her parents. Visiting a qualified health professional can help address these concerns and provide support.

- **Psychosocial Support:**
  - Create safe spaces for girls to discuss menstrual health and related concerns, fostering peer support and mutual understanding.

  - Offer counseling services or support groups for girls experiencing emotional distress or mental health challenges associated with menstruation.

- **Self-Care Practices:**
  - Encourage girls to practice self-care techniques such as regular exercises, stress management, healthy diet and adequate sleep to alleviate symptoms and improve overall wellbeing.

  - Promote the use of relaxation techniques like medication, yoga or deep breathing exercises to reduce stress and manage emotional symptoms.

- **Policy and Advocacy:**
  - Advocate for policies that promote menstrual equity, including access to affordable menstrual products, menstrual hygienic facilities and menstrual leave policies in workplaces and schools if needed.

  - Challenge societal taboos and stigma surrounding menstruation through public awareness campaigns and media representation.

By addressing these challenges systematically through education, access to healthcare, support networks, self-care practices and advocacy efforts, we can better tackle the impact of menarche and menstrual health concerns on adolescent girl's mental health and overall wellbeing.

(B) Development of Secondary Sexual Characters:

- **Thelarche:**
  - o This refers to the first noticeable sign of puberty in the form of breast development, typically occurring between the ages 8 and 13.

  - o Small firm mounds of tissue form under the nipple known as breast buds.

  - o The areola, the pigmented area around the nipple, also enlarges and darkens.

Impact of Breast Development on Mental Health:

  - o **Breast Buds:**
    Development of breast buds can lead to feelings of self-consciousness, body image issues and comparisons with peers.

- **Adrenarche:**

  - o This refers to the activation of adrenal glands, which produce sex hormones like androgens including testosterone.

  - o Adrenarche typically starts around the same time as thelarche, but it can be earlier or later.

  - o Androgen plays crucial role in various pubertal changes including:
    - ✓ Growth of axillary and pubic hairs.

    - ✓ Increased oil production in skin leading to acne.

✓ Deepening of voice.

✓ Development of adult body odour.

✓ Maturation of genetalia.

Impact of Adrenarche on Mental Health:

o **Pubic and Axillary Hairs:**
Growing body hair can cause embarrassment especially if it occurs earlier or later than peers, leading to social stigma and insecurity.

o **Acne:**
Hormonal changes during puberty can trigger acne breakouts, affecting self-esteem and confidence, particularly if severe and persistent.

o **Emotional and Psychological Changes:** Mood swings, increased self-awareness and exploration of identity.

(C) Growth Spurt:

o **Increase in Height:**
A rapid increase in height, often accompanied by changes in body proportions. This growth spurt usually begins around ages 9 – 11 years and peaks around ages 12 – 14, but the timings can vary. On an average, girls gain about 8 – 10 inches (20 – 25 cm) in height during this period. The growth plates in long bones, like those in arms and legs, close towards the end of puberty, signalise the end of significant height increase.

o **Increase in Weight:**
Body weight tends to increase during puberty, partly due to increase in muscle mass and body fat. This weight gain is essential for normal development. Girls often experience changes in body composition, redistributing fat to areas like the hips and breasts, leading to a more curvaceous body shape.

o **Body Contour:**
Puberty brings about changes in body contour as fat distribution alters, resulting in a more defined waistline, broader hips and the development of breasts. These changes are influenced by hormonal fluctuations, particularly estrogen, which plays a significant role in shaping the female body during puberty.

o **Genital Organ Changes:**
  ✓ **Ovaries:** Ovaries change their shape; the elongated shape becomes bulky and oval. The ovarian bulk is due to the follicular enlargement at various stages of development and proliferation of stromal cells.

- ✓ **The Uterine Body and the Cervix:** The ratio at birth is about 1:2, the ratio becomes 1:1 when menarche occurs. Thereafter the enlargement of the body occurs rapidly, so that the ratio soon becomes 2: 1.

- ✓ **The Vaginal Changes:** are more pronounced. A few layers of thin epithelium in a girl becomes stratified epithelium of many layers. They are rich in glycogen due to the effect of estrogen. The Doderlein's bacilli appear which convert glycogen into lactic acid. The vaginal ph becomes acidic, ranging between 4 and 5.

It is important to remember that puberty progresses differently in every girl and it's unique for every girl. The timing and sequence of changes can vary. Some girls may experience all these changes simultaneously, while others may have different intervals between them. If the parents have any concerns about pubertal development of their daughter, they should visit a qualified healthcare professional for further advice.

Impact of Growth Spurt on Mental Health:

- Rapid physical growth can lead to feelings of clumsiness, discomfort and dissatisfaction with one's changing body shape.

- Height disparities with peers can contribute to feelings of self-consciousness, inadequacy or being different.

- **Body Image Concerns:**
  Changes in physical appearance may lead to negative body image perceptions, low self-esteem and increased vulnerability to eating disorders.

- **Social Pressure:**
  Peer comparisons and societal beauty standards can exacerbate feelings of insecurity, isolation and fear of rejection.

- **Emotional Distress:**
  Coping with physical changes and societal expectations may lead to stress, anxiety and depression, affecting overall mental wellbeing.

- **Media Representation:**
  - The media often portrays unrealistic beauty standards, promoting thinness and flawless appearance as the ideal.

  - Images of airbrushed models and celebrities can distort perceptions of normal body shapes and sizes.

  - Constant exposure to edited photos and influenced culture can lead to feelings of inadequacy and self-comparison.

- **Peer Comparison:**
  - Adolescents frequently compare themselves to their peers, striving to meet societal beauty ideal.

  - Peer groups may reinforce certain body standards through comments, jokes or social media interactions.

- **Family Influence:**
  - Family attitudes and behaviors regarding body image can shape adolescent's perception of herself.

  - Negative comments or emphasis on appearance within the family environment can contribute to poor body image.

Strategies to Tackle Challenges during Growth Spurts:

- **Promote Body Positivity:**
  Encourage positive body image by celebrating diverse body shapes and sizes, fostering self-acceptance, and challenging unrealistic beauty ideals.

- **Provide Education:**
  Offer comprehensive sex education that includes information about puberty, body changes and self-care practices to empower girls with knowledge and to reduce stigma.

- **Encourage open communication:**
  Create a supportive environment for girls to express concerns, ask questions and seek guidance from trusted adults, peers or healthcare providers.

- **Foster Peer Support:**
  Facilitate peer support groups or workshops where girls can share their experiences, offer encouragement and build resilience together.

- **Emphasize Self-care:**
  Teach self-care practices such as proper hygiene, skincare routines, healthy eating habits and regular exercise to promote physical and mental wellbeing.

- **Provide Access to resources:**
  Ensure access to healthcare services, mental health support and resources for managing acne, body hairs and other physical changes.

- **Challenge Stereotypes:**
  Counteract stereotypes and stigma surrounding puberty and adolescent development through education, advocacy and media representation.

- **Promote Positive Coping Strategies:**
  Teach coping skills such as mindfulness, stress management techniques, creative outlets and positive self-talk to help girls navigate changes and build resilience.

- **Media Literacy:**
  o Educate adolescents about media literacy and the ways in which images are often digitally altered.

  o Encourage critical thinking and skepticism towards media representation of beauty.

- **Body Positivity:**
  o Promote body positivity and acceptance of diverse body shapes and sizes.

- o Highlight the value of health and wellbeing over appearance.

- **Healthy Habits:**
  - o Encourage healthy habits such as regular exercise, balanced nutrition and adequate sleep for overall wellbeing.

  - o Emphasize the importance of self-care and self-compassion.

- **Positive Self-Talk:**
  - o Teach adolescents to recognize and challenge negative self-talk and internalized criticism.

  - o Encourage affirmations and positive self-statements to cultivate self-compassion.

- **Diverse Role Models:**
  - o Provide exposure to diverse role models who challenge traditional beauty norms and celebrate authenticity.

  - o Highlight achievements and talents beyond physical appearance.

- **Open Communication:**
  - o Foster open communication within families and peer groups about body image and self-esteem.

  - o Create a supportive environment where adolescents feel comfortable discussing their concerns and seeking support.

- **Limit Social Media Exposure:**
  - Encourage adolescents to limit their exposure to social media and unfollow accounts that promote unrealistic beauty standards.

  - Emphasize the importance of cultivating real-life relationships and hobbies outside of digital world.

By addressing these changes systematically through education, support networks, self-care practices and promoting positive coping strategies, we can help adolescent girls navigate the developmental changes of puberty more confidently and maintain better mental health and wellbeing.

(D) The Risk-taking behaviours in Adolescent Girls:

The risk-taking behaviors in Adolescent Girls related to substance abuse, self-harm and risky sexual behavior and resources for seeking help:

Substance Abuse:

- Experimentation with drugs or alcohol as a means of coping with stress, peer pressure or curiosity.

- Consequences may include addiction, impaired cognitive function, physical health problems, academic or legal issues and strained relationships with family and peers.

- **Resources for seeking help include:**
  - School counselors or nurses who can provide support and guidance.

  - Substance abuse hotlines or helplines or confidential assistance.

  - Rehabilitation centers or outpatient programs specializing in substance abuse treatment.

Self-harm:

- Engaging in self-harm behaviors such as cutting, burning or hitting oneself as a way to cope with emotional pain or distress.

- Consequences may include physical injury, scarring, infection, worsening mental health symptoms and potential escalation of self-harm behaviors.

- **Resources for seeking help include:**
    o Mental health professionals such as therapists, counselors or psychiatrists who can provide therapy and support.

    o Crisis hotlines or helplines staffed by trained professionals who can offer immediate assistance and referral to appropriate services.

    o Support groups or online communities for individuals struggling with self-harm to connect with others and share experiences.

Risky Sexual Behavior:

- Engaging in unprotected sex, multiple sexual partners or sexual activity under the influence of drugs or alcohol.

- Consequences may include unintended pregnancy, sexually transmitted infections (STIs), emotional trauma, relationship conflicts and social stigma.

- **Resources for seeking help include:**
    o Sexual help clinics or Planned Parenthood Centers for confidential STIs testing, contraception and reproductive health services.

    o School counselors or nurses who can provide education on safe sex practices and referrals to appropriate resources.

    o Mental health professionals who specialize in sexual health and relationships and who can offer support and guidance in navigating sexual decision-making.

In each case it is crucial for adolescent girls to understand the potential consequences of these risk-taking behaviors and to seek help from trusted adults or professional resources when needed. Engaging open communication and reducing stigma surrounding these issues can help adolescents feel more comfortable seeking support and accessing necessary resources for their wellbeing.

(E) Role of Family Relationships in Adolescent Mental Health:

Role of family relationships in adolescent mental health, addressing parental expectations, conflict in family unit and how to take advice support from trusted adults:

Parental Expectations:

- Parents often have expectations regarding their child's academic performance, career choices and behavior.

- Unrealistic or excessive parental expectations can contribute to stress, anxiety and feelings of inadequacy in adolescents.

- Pressure to meet parental expectations may lead to conflicts and strained relationships within family.

Conflicts within the Family Unit:

- Conflicts within the family, such as disagreement between parents, sibling rivalry or communication breakdowns can impact adolescent mental health.

- Hostile or dysfunctional family dynamics may contribute to feelings of insecurity, anxiety or depression in adolescents.

- Exposure to parental conflict or divorce/separation can further exacerbate mental health issues and emotional distress.

Taking Advice and Support from Trusted Adults:

- Identify trusted adults within your support network such as parents, relatives, teachers or mentors who can provide guidance and support.

- Foster open and honest communication with trusted adults, expressing your concerns, feelings and need in a respectful manner.

- Seek advice and support from trusted adults when facing challenges or making important decisions such as academic choices, peer conflicts or personal struggles.

- Be receptive to feedback and guidance from trusted adults, even it may differ from your initial perspective or preferences.

- Collaborate with trusted adults to explore potential solutions, coping strategies and resources for managing stressors and improving mental wellbeing.

By acknowledging the role of family relationships in adolescent mental health, addressing parental expectations and conflicts within the family unit and seeking advice and support from trusted adults, adolescents can navigate challenges more effectively and foster healthier relationships within their family and support network.

(F) Causes for Adolescent Girls to Become Emotionally
Unstable:

Causes for adolescent girls to become emotionally unstable and how to normalize mental health issues in adolescent girls with the help of resources:

Causes for Adolescent Girls to Become Emotionally Unstable:

- **Hormonal Changes:**
  Fluctuations in hormones during puberty can lead to mood swings, irritability and emotional instability in adolescent girls.

- **Stress and Pressure:**
  Academic pressure, social expectations, family conflicts and peer relationships can contribute to stress and overwhelm, leading to emotional instability.

- **Social Media Influence:**
  Constant exposure to curated and filtered images on social media platforms can create unrealistic expectations and lead to feelings of inadequacy and low-esteem.

- **Trauma and Adversity:**
  Experiences of trauma, such as abuse, neglect or loss can have a profound impact on adolescent mental health and emotional stability.

- **Mental Health Disorders:**
  Adolescent girls may experience mental health disorders, which can manifest as emotional instability or through genetically inherited.

How to Normalize Mental Health Issues in Adolescent Girls with the Help of Resources:

Maintain a Positive Mindset:

- Embrace change as an opportunity for growth and self-discovery, rather than viewing it as a source of stress and uncertainty.

- Cultivate resilience by focusing on your strengths, adaptability and ability to overcome challenges.

Stay Flexible and Open-Minded:

- Be willing to adapt to new circumstances, routines and expectations and change your approach with an open mind and willingness to learn.

- Be proactive in seeking out resources, support and opportunities for personal and academic growth.

Education and Awareness:

- Provide education and information about the mental health to adolescents, families and school communities to reduce stigma and increase understanding.

- Normalize discussions about mental health by integrating it into school curricula, assemblies and awareness campaigns.

- Offer resources such as books such as this, articles and online platforms that provide reliable information and support for mental health issues.

School Counselors:

- School counselors pay a crucial role in supporting the mental health of adolescent girls by providing counseling, resources and referrals to appropriate services.

- Encourage students to utilize the services of school counselors for confidential support, guidance and assistance with mental health concerns.

- Collaborate with school counselors to implement mental health programs, workshops or support groups that address the specific needs of adolescent girls.

Support Groups:

- Learn on trusted adults such as parents, teachers, mentors or counselors for advice, encouragement and support during times of transition.

- Don't hesitate to ask for help or seek professional guidance if you are struggling to cope with change or experiencing emotional difficulties.

- Support groups provide a sense of community understanding and solidarity for adolescents experiencing similar mental health challenges.

- Encourage adolescents to join support groups focused on topics such as anxiety, depression, self-esteem or body image.

- Facilitate connections with peer support networks online or in-person where adolescents can share experiences, offer encouragement and receive validation and support.

Open Communication within Families:

- Foster an environment of open communication within families where discussions about emotions, struggles and mental health are welcomed and normalized.

- Encourage parents to actively listen to their adolescent daughters, validate their feelings and offer support without judgement.

- Model healthy communication and coping strategies within the family and prioritize empathy, understanding and respect in interactions with one another.

Peer Education and Support:

- Empower adolescent girls to become mental health advocates and peer supporters within their schools and communities.

- Train student leaders or peer mentors to facilitate discussions, workshops or awareness campaigns on mental health topics and resources.

- Create peer support networks or buddy systems where adolescents can lean on one another for emotional support and encouragement.

Time Management:

- Break tasks into smaller manageable chunks and prioritize them based on importance and deadlines.

- Use tools such as planners or digital calendars to organize schedules and set realistic goals.

- Allocate time for self-care activities and relaxation to prevent burn out.

Develop Healthy Boundaries:

- Identify your personal boundaries and communicate them with your friends.

- Set limits and time and energy you invest in friendships and prioritize self-care and personal wellbeing.

Recognize Red Flags:

- Be aware of signs of unhealthy relationships, such as manipulation, jealousy and disrespect.

- Trust your instincts and distance yourself from toxic and negative influences.

Balance Online and Offline Interactions:

- Limit time spent on social media and cultivate real life relationships through face-to-face interactions.

- Be mindful of the impact of social media on your mental health and curate your online environment to promote positivity and authenticity.

Deep Breathing Exercises:

- Practice deep breathing exercises to promote relaxation and reduce stress. Techniques such as diaphragmatic breathing can help regulate emotions and calm the nervous system.

- Incorporate deep breathing exercises into daily routines such as before bedtime or during moments of heightened stress or anxiety.

Seeking Professional Help:

- If emotional instability persists or significantly impacts daily functioning, seek professional help from a therapist, counselor or mental health professional.

- A mental health professional can provide individualized assessment, support and evidence-based interventions to address underlying issues and develop coping strategies.

- Therapists offer specialized mental health treatment and support for adolescents experiencing a range of issues, including anxiety, depression, trauma and behavioral challenges.

- Therapy modalities such as cognitive-behavior therapy (CBT), dialectical behavior therapy (DBT) or mindfulness-based interventions can be effective in managing emotional instability and improving overall wellbeing.

- Encourage adolescents and families to seek therapy when needed and provide information about how to find a therapist who has specialized in the field.

- Normalize the idea of therapy as valuable research for personal growth, self-discovery and emotional wellbeing.

By addressing the underlying causes of emotional instability, practicing deep breathing exercises and seeking professional help when needed, adolescent girls can learn to manage their emotions effectively and improve their overall mental health and wellbeing.

By approaching transitions with a proactive and positive mindset, seeking support when needed and staying resilient in the phase of challenges; adolescents can navigate these milestones successfully and thrive in their academic, personal and professional pursuits.

By normalizing mental health issues through education, access to resources such as school counselors and therapist's participation in support groups and fostering open communication within families and communities, we can create a culture of acceptance, support and resilience for adolescent girls facing mental health challenges.

CHAPTER III: CHILD MARRIAGES AND ITS IMPACT ON GIRL'S MENTAL HEALTH

(A) Definition of Child Marriage:

Child marriage, defined as marriage before the age of 18, has severe and far-reaching impact on mental health of adolescent girls. This harmful practice is prevalent in many parts of the world, especially in regions with high poverty levels, limited access to education and traditional norms that undervalue the role of girls and women.

(B) Magnitude of the Problem:

Child marriage remains a significant global issue, affecting millions of girls each year, with particularly high prevalence in certain regions, including South Asia and Sub-Saharan Africa.

UNICEF (May 2023 Global Update):

- An estimated 640 million girls and women alive today were married in childhood.

- Nearly half of child brides live in Asia (45%) with the next largest share in sub-Saharan Africa (20%), followed by East Asia and the Pacific (15%) and Latin America and the Caribbean (9%).

- India alone accounts for one third of the world's child brides.

- Child marriages has declined steadily in South Asia, but little progress has been seen in many other parts of the world. The global prevalence of child marriage has fallen from 23% to 19% in last 10 years.

- Across all regions, progress in child marriage has primarily benefitted girls from the richest families.

- **Looking Ahead to Eliminating Child Marriage:**

  o Declining in the levels of child marriages are not occurring at a fast enough pace to reach the SDG target of ***"Eliminating the Practice By 2030."***

  o Ending Child Marriage is an ambitious global target and as per the available data, it is not within easy reach by 2030. To spare girls from this violation of rights, efforts to accelerate progress need to be 20 times faster than the present.

  o Ending child marriage is an obligation, necessary to secure the rights of girls around the world.

Indian Scenario:

- **Prevalence:**
  India accounts for a significant portion of the world's child brides, with about 223 million child brides, the highest number globally. About 1 in 3 of the world's child brides live in India.

- **Regional Variations:**
  There is considerable variation across Indian States. For example, states like Bihar, West Bengal and Rajasthan have higher rates of child marriage, while states in the southern and northern regions generally have lower rates.

- **Child Marriage Act in India:**

  o **Historical Background:**
  - The Child Marriage Restraint Act, 1929 (Sarda Act):
    The first legislature in India aimed at curbing child marriage was the Child Marriage Restraint Act, commonly known as the Sarda Act, passed in 1929. It set the minimum age of marriage at 14 for girls and 18 for boys. The act was a significant step forward but had limited impact due to weak enforcement and societal acceptance of child marriage.

  - **Amendments and Developments:**
    The Act was amended in 1949 and 1978, raising the minimum marriageable age for girls to 15 and then to 18, and for boys to 21.

  - Despite these amendments, enforcement remained weak, and child marriages continued to be prevalent, especially in rural areas.

- o **Provision of Child Marriage Act (PCMA), 2006:**
  - The Provision of Child Marriage Act, 2006, was enacted to address the limitations of the previous law. The Act sets the legal marriage age at 18 for girls and 21 for boys and explicitly prohibits the solemnization of child marriages.

  - Despite the legal framework, enforcement remains a significant challenge. Many child marriages go unreported due to the reluctance of families, social norms and lack of awareness.

  - *In many communities, child marriage is still culturally accepted, making it difficult to implement the law effectively.*

- o **Progress in Reducing Child Marriage:**
  - **Decline in Prevalence:** There has been noticeable decline in the prevalence of child marriage in India over the past decades. According to the National Family Health Survey (NFHS), the percentage of women aged 20 – 24 who were married before the age of 18 decreased from 47% in 2005-06 (NFHS-3) to around 23% in 2019-21 (NFHS-5). This represents a significant reduction in certain states and communities.

  - **Role of Education:** Increased access to education for girls has been a crucial factor in reducing child marriages. Girls who stay in school longer are less likely to be married at a younger age.

- o **Government Initiatives:**
  - The Indian Government has launched several initiatives to combat child marriages, such as **"Beti Bachav Beti Padhav Campaign"**, which

focuses on the empowerment of girls through education and awareness.

- Schemes like the **"Kanyashree Prakalpa"** in West Bengal provide financial incentives to delay marriage and continue education.

o **Civil Society Efforts:**
NGOs and civil society organizations have played a critical role in raising awareness, providing education and supporting victims of child marriage. There grassroots work has contributed to changing societal attitudes towards child marriage.

o **Comparative Progress:**
- **Regional Differences:** While the overall trend shows a decline, the progress is uneven across different regions in India. States like Kerala and Tamil Nadu have made significant strides in reducing child marriage, while states like Bihar, West Bengal and Rajasthan continue to report higher rates.

- **Urban vs Rural:** Urban areas generally have lower rates of child marriages compared to rural areas, where traditional practices and economic pressures are more prevalent.

- **Ongoing Challenges:** Despite progress, challenges such as poverty, gender inequality, lack of education and social norms continue to perpetuate child marriage in certain areas. The COVID-19 pandemic has also led to a resurgence in child marriages in some regions due to economic hardships and school closures.

The Prohibition of Child Marriage Act, 2006 represents a significant legislative step towards eradicating child marriages in India. While progress has been made in reducing the prevalence of child marriages, especially in urban areas and among educated communities, the practice still persists in various part of country. Addressing the child marriages in India requires a multifaceted approach that goes beyond legal measures. It involves changing deep-seated cultural norms, improving access to education, empowering girls and providing economic support to families. Collaboration between government, civil societies and communities is crucial to create a society where every girl can grow up free from the threat of early marriage.

(C) Impact of Child Marriages on Mental Health:

1. Psychological Trauma:

- **Early Sexual Activity:**
  Girls who marry young are often subjected to early sexual activity, frequently without their consent, leading to trauma, depression and anxiety.

- **Domestic Violence:**
  Child brides are more likely to experience domestic violence, which can result in long-lasting psychological damage, including post-traumatic stress disorder (PTSD).

- **Isolation:**
  Many girls are isolated from their families and peers after marriage, contributing to feelings of loneliness and depression.

2. Loss of Adolescence:

- **Interruption of Education:**
  Child marriage often results in the abrupt end of a girl's education, depriving her opportunities for personal and intellectual growth, leading to feelings of inadequacy and hopelessness.

- **Burden of Adult Responsibilities:**
  Young brides are thrown into adult roles and responsibilities, such as child bearing and managing a household, before they are emotionally or physically prepared, increasing stress and anxiety.

3. Long-term Mental Health Consequences:

- **Depression and Anxiety:**
  The pressures and traumas associated with child marriage can lead to long-term mental health issues, including chronic depression and anxiety disorders.

- **Self-Esteem Issues:**
  The lack of autonomy and control over their lives can severely affect the self-esteem and self-worth of these girls, leading to diminished sense of identity.

- **Suicidal Thoughts and Behavior:**
  The combination of abuse, behavior and lack of support can push some child brides towards suicidal thoughts and behaviors.

4. Impact on Motherhood:

- **Maternal Mental Health:**
  Young mothers, often still children themselves, are at a higher risk for postpartum depression and other mental health issues related to the challenges of motherhood.

- **Intergenerational Trauma:**
  The mental health issue experienced by child brides can also affect their ability to provide a supportive environment for their children, perpetuating a cycle of trauma and mental health issues across generations.

The mental health impacts of child marriage are profound and multifaceted, affecting adolescent girls' emotional well-being, development and future potential. Addressing child marriage requires a holistic approach that includes legal reforms, education, empowerment of girls and accessible mental health support to mitigate the damage and prevent the continuation of this harmful practice.

CHAPTER IV: MENTAL HEALTH IN REPRODUCTIVE YEARS

"Your strength and resilience

create the foundation for the future."

Motherhood is a transformative journey that brings joy, challenges and profound changes to a woman's life. Amid the joyous moment and new beginning, it is essential to acknowledge the less discussed aspects of motherhood, particularly those related to mental health.

The transition to motherhood is marked by hormonal fluctuations, sleep deprivation and adjustment to a new role, potentially impacting a women's mental wellbeing.

The journey through motherhood, especially when complicated by delayed marriages due to carrier opportunities, infertility, abortions or bad obstetric history and further exacerbated by the pursuit of IVF and its financial implications; can significantly impact a woman's mental health.

The transition from adulthood to motherhood is a potentially vulnerable time for some women's mental health and approximately 9 – 21% of women experience depression and anxiety at this time. Many more experience subclinical symptoms of depression and/or anxiety, stress, low esteem and loss of confidence.

Postpartum mental disorders, including postpartum depression, anxiety disorders and even rare but severe cases of postpartum psychosis; can throw a shadow over this joyous moment of being mother.

In reproductive years, impact on women's mental health can be addressed in different stages including selecting a perfect life partner, preparing and navigating the journey of motherhood, postpartum mental health, balancing career, family and parental responsibilities.

(A) Unique Challenges for Girls in Selecting Life Partner and its impact on mental health:

- **Social Expectations:**
  Girls often face societal pressure to find a partner who meets certain criteria such as financial stability, social status and family background. The fear of not meeting these expectations can lead to stress and anxiety.

- **Double Standards:**
  Girls may encounter double standards regarding their partner choices, facing criticism or judgement for being too pinky or too lenient. This can create confusion and self-doubt, affecting their mental wellbeing.

- **Gender Stereotypes:**
  Gender role and stereotypes can influence partner selection, with girls feeling pressure to find a partner who conforms to traditional masculine ideals. Straying from these norms may result in social backlash and internal conflicts.

- **Cultural and Religious Factors:**
  Cultural and religious beliefs often play a significant role in partner selection. Girls may experience conflicts between personal desires and familiar

expectations leading to feelings of guilt and identity crisis.

- **Fear of Rejection and Failure:**
  The fear of rejection and choosing a wrong partner can be overwhelming for girls, impacting their self-esteem and confidence. This fear may stem from past experiences of societal messages about the consequences of failed relationships.

- **Balancing Personal and Partner Goals:**
  Girls may struggle to balance their own aspirations with those of their potential partner, particularly if they feel pressurized to prioritize the needs of the relationship over their own. This can lead to feelings of resentment and dissatisfaction.

- **Lack of Agency and Autonomy:**
  In some cultures, and families, girls may have limited autonomy in choosing their life partner, leading to feeling of helplessness and frustration. This lack of agency can have long-term effects on mental health including low self-worth and depression.

- **Financial Dependence:**
  Economic factors can influence partner selection, with girls feeling pressured to choose a partner who can provide financial stability. This dependency on a partner for financial security can impact mental wellbeing if the relationship becomes strained.

- **Intergenerational Conflicts:**
  General differences in values and expectations can create tension when selecting a life partner. Girls may struggle to navigate conflicting opinions from older

family members while staying true to their own desires, leading to stress and emotional turmoil.

Systematic Approach to Counter or to Deal with Challenges in Selecting Life Partner:

- **Self-awareness and Clarification of Needs:**
  Encourage the girl to reflect on her values, goals and preferences in her life partner. This self-awareness will guide her in selecting someone compatible.

- **Open Communication:**
  Family members and friends can create a supportive environment where the girl feels comfortable discussing her concerns and preferences openly.

- **Education and Awareness:**
  Provide information about healthy relationships, red flags to watch for and the importance of mutual respect and communication.

- **Encourage Healthy Boundaries:**
  Help her establish and maintain healthy boundaries in relationships, teaching her to prioritize her own wellbeing and happiness.

- **Empower Decision-Making:**
  Support her in making her own choices rather than imposing expectations or judgements. Encourage her to trust her instincts.

- **Access to Resources:**
  Provide access to resources such as relationship counseling, books or workshops that can offer

guidance and support in navigating the complexities of relationships.

- **Encourage Independence:**
  Foster her independence and self-insufficiency, reminding her that she doesn't need to rely solely on a partner for fulfillment and happiness.

- **Promote Self-Care:**
  Encourage the girl to prioritize self-care activities that promote and emotional wellbeing such as exercise, hobbies and spending time with supporting friends and families.

- **Normalize Seeking Help:**
  Remove the stigma around seeking help from mental health professionals if needed. Let her know it is okay to seek support and guidance from a therapist or counselor.

- **Monitor Mental Health:**
  Keep an eye on her mental health and wellbeing, checking in regularly to see how she is coping with relationship challenges and offering support as needed.

With this approach, a girl can navigate the challenges of selecting a life partner with support from family, friends and mental health professionals, minimizing the impact on her mental health.

(B) Impact on Mental Health of a Woman while Navigating through Motherhood:

Navigating through motherhood can pose significant challenges to a woman's mental health, especially when facing delays in conceiving due to carrier opportunities, infertility, repeated abortions and/or a bad obstetric history leading to pursuit of IVF (In-Vitro-Fertilization) and the associated financial burden.

Delay in Conceiving Due to Career Opportunities:

The best age to marry a girl, or anyone for that matter is a highly individual and subjective matter that can vary depending on personal circumstances, cultural norms and individual preferences. There is no **"one size fits-all answer"** to this question as people mature and develop at different rates, have different life goals and face different challenges.

It is important to note that marriage is a significant life decision that should not be rushed into. Factors such as emotional maturity, financial stability, readiness for commitment, compatibility with the partner and personal goals should all be taken into consideration when deciding for right time for marriage.

Dr. Fisher believes that marriages that take place when the couple is in their late 20s and mid 30s are most successful. "By the time we are getting to late 20s, we have a clear sense of who we are and what we want out of life," he explains.

But this trend is changing in recent years with people choosing to marry later in life for various reasons such as pursuing education, personal goals and personal development and may land in:

- Feelings of frustration, anxiety or guilt about postponing motherhood for pursuing education, carrier later in life.

- There can be pressure from societal expectations or family members to prioritize either carrier or motherhood.

Infertility:

Pregnancy and child-bearing are key life events and studies have shown the happiness of mother, the couple as a whole before, during and after childbirth.

Some believe that pregnancy can make you aware of the world around you and that preparing for the baby can make you feel more secure and confident. Family members often treat you well when they hear you are pregnant.

Inability to conceive naturally can cause feelings of shame, guilt and low self-esteem. These negative feelings may lead varying degrees of depression, anxiety, distress and a poor quality of life.

Studies have shown that infertile couples experience significant anxiety and emotional distress, when fertility treatment proves to be unsuccessful, for instance, women and couples can experience deep feelings of grief and loss.

Infertility can lead to:

- Emotional distress including feelings of inadequacy, sadness or despair.

- Strain on relationships, as fertility can cause tension between partners.

- Social isolation such as interaction with friends or family members without children may become difficult.

- Loss of self-esteem and identity tied to traditional notions of womanhood or motherhood.

Repeated Abortions can lead to:

- Psychological trauma, including guilt, shame or grief.

- Fear of future pregnancies and anxieties about potential complications.

- Impact on mental wellbeing, potentially leading to depression or anxiety disorders.

Bad Obstetric History can lead to:

- PTSD (Post-Traumatic Stress Disorder) symptoms due to traumatic childbirth experiences.

- Anxiety and fear surrounding subsequent pregnancies or childbirth.

- Grief and mourning for lost pregnancies or children.

In-Vitro Fertilization (IVF) and Financial Burden can lead to:

- Stress and anxiety related to the IVF process, including hormonal treatments, injections and medical procedures.

- Financial strain from the high costs of IVF, leading to worries about financial instability.

- Feelings of guilt or pressure to justify the financial investment, especially when unsuccessful even with IVF.

- Impact on overall wellbeing, as financial stressors can exacerbate existing mental health issues.

How to Tackle the Impact on Mental Health for a Woman Navigating through Motherhood.

Seeking Professional Support:

- Encourage women to seek support from mental health professionals such as therapists or counselors, who specialize in fertility issues and maternal mental health.

- Provide information about support groups or online communities where women can connect with others who have experienced similar challenges.

Open Communication:

- Encourage open communication between partners to share feelings, concerns and expectations about the journey to parenthood.

- Facilitate discussions about coping strategies, including how to manage stress and anxiety together.

Education and Information:

- Offer education about fertility, reproductive health and the IVF process to empower the women with knowledge and understanding.

- Provide resources and information about potential risks, challenges and success rates associated with IVF treatment.

Emotional Support:

- Offer emotional support to address feelings of grief, loss or disappointment related to delayed conception and bad obstetric history.

- Validate the women's emotions and provide a safe space for her to express her feelings without judgement.

Self-Care Practices:

- Encourage self-care practices such as mindfulness, relaxation techniques, exercise and hobbies to help manage stress and promote overall wellbeing.

- Emphasize the importance of self-compassion and self-kindness throughout the journey.

Building a Support Network:

- Encourage the woman to build a strong support network of friends, family and healthcare professionals who can offer practical and emotional support.

- Provide resources for connecting with other women who have experienced similar challenges through support groups or online forums.

Addressing Financial Concerns:

- Offer guidance on financial planning and resources for managing the financial burden of IVF treatment, such as exploring insurance coverage, grants or financial assistance programs.

- Help women develop a budget and explore alternative options for financing treatment of infertility, if needed.

Regular Check-ups and Monitoring:

- Schedule regular check-ups with healthcare providers to monitor emotional wellbeing, provides updates on treatment progress and address any concerns or questions.

- Monitor for signs of depression, anxiety or other mental health issues and provide appropriate interventions or referrals as needed.

By following these approaches, women can successfully navigate through motherhood or even through infertility, and if no success in IVF treatment, then by going for adoption.

(C) Postpartum Mental Disorders:

Postpartum mental disorders are mental illnesses that can occur after child birth and can negatively impact the mother, the infant and the family as a whole.

Postpartum mental health disorders are a significant concern worldwide, with varying prevalence rates influenced by a multitude of factors.

In India, the high prevalence of postpartum mental health disorders is influenced by socio-economic disparities, cultural stigmas and inadequate mental health infrastructure. Increasing awareness, improving healthcare services and promoting mental health education are crucial for addressing these issues.

Three main types of postpartum mental disorders include:

- Postpartum Blues

- Postpartum Depression

- Postpartum Psychosis

Predisposing Factors for Postpartum Mental Disorders

Biological Factors:

- **Hormonal Changes:**
  Significant fluctuations in estrogen and progesterone levels after childbirth. Estrogen and Progesterone levels suddenly drops significantly.

- **Genetic Predisposition:**
  Family history of depression, anxiety or other mental health disorders.

- **Medical Complications:**
  Complications during pregnancy or childbirth, for example preeclampsia, emergency C-Section etc.

- **Sleep Deprivation:**
  Chronic lack of sleep due to prolonged labor and newborn care.

Psychological Factors:

- **Personal History of Mental Issues:**
  Previous episodes of depression, anxiety, or other psychiatric conditions.

- **Personality Traits:**
  High levels of neuroticism, low self-esteem and high levels of perfectionism.

- **Stress and Anxiety:**
  High levels of prenatal stress and anxiety.

- **Unrealistic Expectations:**
  Unrealistic expectation about motherhood and the postpartum period.

Social Factors:

- **Lack of Social Support:**
  Limited support from family, friends and community.

- **Marital or Relationship Problems:**
  Conflicts or dissatisfaction in relationships.

- **Socio-economic Status:**
  Low income, financial stress and unstable housing.

- **Cultural Factors:**
  Cultural stigmas surrounding mental health and motherhood.

- **Isolation:**
  Physical or emotional isolation from support networks.

Environmental Factors:

- **Stressful Life Events:**
  Recent significant life changes or traumas, for example loss of a loved one or job loss.

- **Living Conditions:**
  Poor living conditions or a stressful home environment.

- **Work- Related Stress:**
  Balancing work and new motherhood, lack of maternity leave or job security.

Obstetric Factors:

- **Complicated pregnancy or delivery:**
  Experiences such as preterm birth, birth trauma or neonatal complications.

- **Unplanned or Unwanted Pregnancy:**
  Lack of preparedness or ambivalence about the pregnancy.

Infant-Related Factors:

- **Infant Health Issues:**
  Health problems or special needs in the newborn.

- **Breastfeeding Issues:**
  Difficulties in breastfeeding, which can affect maternal mood.

Postpartum mental disorders result from a complex interplay of biological, psychological, social, environmental, obstetric and infant-related factors. Understanding these predisposing factors can help in early identification, prevention and intervention strategies to support maternal mental health.

Postpartum Blues:

Definition:

Postpartum blues also known as "baby blues", refer to a transient mood disturbance experienced by mothers shortly after childbirth. It is characterized by mild depressive symptoms and emotional instability but is generally not as severe as postpartum depression.

Prevalence:

Postpartum blues are common, affecting up to 70 – 80% of new mothers. Symptoms typically begins within first few days postpartum and can last for up to two weeks.

Symptomatology:

Symptoms of postpartum blues include:

- Mood swings
- Anxiety
- Irritability
- Tearfulness
- Sadness
- Insomnia
- Fatigue
- Difficulty in concentrating
- Feeling overwhelmed

These symptoms are usually mild and self-limiting.

Pathophysiology;

The exact pathophysiology is not fully understood, but several factors contribute to its development.

- **Hormonal Changes:**
  The rapid decline in estrogen and progesterone levels following delivery is believed to play a crucial role. These hormones which increase significantly during pregnancy, drop sharply after childbirth, potentially affecting neurotransmitter regulation and mood stability.

- **Neurotransmitter Dysregulation:**
  Hormonal changes may influence the levels and activity of neurotransmitters like serotonin, dopamine and norepinephrine. These neurotransmitters are involved in mood regulation and their imbalance can lead to mood disturbances.

- **Stress and Fatigue:**
  The physical and emotional stress of childbirth combined with the demands of caring for a newborn, can contribute feelings of exhaustion, overwhelm and mood swings. Sleep deprivation is also a significant factor, as it can adversely affect emotional wellbeing.

- **Psychosocial Factors:**
  Emotional and social factors such as adjustment to new parental roles, changes in relationships and concerns about infant care, can also influence mood. The support system available to the new mother, including family and community support, plays a crucial role in mitigating or exacerbating symptoms.

- **Genetic and biological vulnerability:**
  Some women may have a genetic predisposition or pre-existing vulnerability to mood disorders, which can be triggered or exacerbated by childbirth and the associated hormonal shifts.

- **Inflammatory Responses:**
  Emerging research suggests that inflammation and immune system changes occurring in postpartum period, may also contribute to mood disturbances. Childbirth can trigger inflammatory process, which might affect brain function and mood.

Diagnosis:

Diagnosis of postpartum blues is clinical and based on the presence of characteristic symptoms occurring within the first two weeks after childbirth. It is important to differentiate postpartum blues from postpartum depression and other psychiatric disorders.

Prognosis:

The prognosis for postpartum blues is generally good. Symptoms usually resolve on their own within two weeks postpartum without specific treatment. If symptoms persist beyond this period, it may indicate the onset of postpartum depression, requiring further evaluation.

Complications:

While postpartum blues themselves do not lead to serious complications, they can increase the risk of developing postpartum depression. It is important to monitor mothers for any worsening of symptoms or prolonged emotional distress.

Management:

Postpartum blues are generally transient and resolve on their own without medical intervention.

Management of postpartum blues primarily involves:

- **Reassurance and Support:**
  Providing reassurance that postpartum blues are common and usually temporary. Emotional support from family and friends is crucial.

- **Education:**
  Informing the mother about the condition and normalizing her experiences.

- **Rest and Self-Care:**
  Encouraging adequate rest, nutrition and self-care.

- **Social Support:**
  Ensuring that the mother has access to social support networks and community resources.

- **Monitoring:**
  Keeping an eye on the severity and duration of symptoms to identify any signs of postpartum depression early.

If symptoms persist or worsens, referral to a healthcare provider for further evaluation and possible treatment of postpartum depression or other mental health conditions is necessary.

Postpartum Depression (PPD):

Definition:

Postpartum depression is a severe long-lasting mood disorder that can affect women after giving birth to the baby. It can affect women after childbirth, surrogates and adoptive parents, though it is commonly associated with biological mothers. PPD is characterized by severe emotional, physical and behavioral changes that interfere with the care of the new born and also day-to-day activities.

Prevalence:

Postpartum depression affects approximately 10 – 20% of new mothers worldwide, although prevalence rates can vary based on cultural, socio-economic and healthcare factors. It is less commonly diagnosed in fathers with prevalence rate ranging from 1 – 10%.

Symptomatology:

Symptoms of postpartum depression are similar to those of major depression but occurs within the first year after childbirth. Symptoms include:

- Persistent sadness or depressed mood.
- Severe mood swings
- Excessive crying
- Difficulty in bonding with the baby.
- Withdrawal from family and friends
- Loss of appetite or eating much more than usual diet.
- Insomnia or sleeping too much.
- Overwhelming fatigue or loss of energy.

- Reduced interest and pleasure in activities once enjoyed.
- Intense irritability and anger
- Feelings of worthlessness, shame, guilt or inadequacy.
- Difficulty in concentrating and making decisions.
- Severe anxiety and panic attacks.
- Thoughts of harming oneself or the baby.

Pathophysiology:

The exact cause of postpartum depression not entirely understood, but it is believed to result from a combination of hormonal, genetic, psychological and environmental factors.

- **Hormonal Changes:**
  After childbirth, there is a significant drop in estrogen and progesterone levels, which may trigger depression in some women.

- **Genetic Factors:**
  A family history of depression or other mood disorders can increase the risk.

- **Psychosocial Stressors:**
  Lack of support, marital problems, financial stress and a history of stress and a history of trauma or abuse can contribute to the development of PPD.

- **Biological Factors:**
  Changes in thyroid function and levels of other hormones such as cortisol may also play a role.

Diagnosis:

Diagnosing postpartum depression involves a comprehensive evaluation by a healthcare provider (Psychiatrists), which may include:

- **Clinical Interviews:**
  Discussing symptoms, thoughts, feelings and overall mental health history.

- **Screening Tools:**
  Using standardized questionnaire such as **the Edinburgh Postnatal Depression Scale (EPDS) or the Patient Health Questionaire-9 (PHQ-9).**

- **Physical Exam:**
  Conducting a physical exam to rule out other causes of symptoms.

- **Laboratory Tests:**
  Checking for thyroid dysfunction or other medical conditions that could contribute to depressive symptoms.

Prognosis:

With appropriate treatment, the prognosis for postpartum depression is generally good. Many women recover fully, especially with early intervention. However, if left untreated, PPD can last for months or even years and may affect the mother's ability to make bonding with her baby and also to perform day-to-day activities.

Complications:

If untreated, postpartum depression can lead to several complications.

- Chronic depression or recurrence of major depressive episodes.

- Impaired mother-infant bonding and attachment issues.

- Developmental delays in the child.

- Increased risk of substance abuse.

- Strained relationships with family members.

- Increased risk of maternal suicide or infanticide (in severe cases).

Management:

Management of postpartum depression typically involves a combination of therapies.

- **Psychotherapy:**
  Cognitive behavioral therapy (CBT) and **interventional therapy (IVT)** are particularly effective. Therapy can help address negative thought patterns, improve coping skills and strengthen social support networks.

- **Medication:**
  Antidepressants such as selective serotonin reuptake inhibitors (SSRIs), can be prescribed, especially for moderate to severe cases. Breastfeeding

considerations are important when selecting medications.

- **Support Groups:**
Joining support groups for new parents can provide a sense of community and shared experiences.

- **Lifestyle Changes:**
Regular physical activity, adequate sleep, healthy eating and mindfulness practices can overall improve mental health.

- **Hospitalization:**
In severe cases, hospitalization may be necessary to ensure the safety of the mother and baby.

Early identification and intervention are crucial for the effective management of postpartum depression, helping to ensure the health and wellbeing of both the mother and the child.

Postpartum Psychosis:

Postpartum psychosis is a severe mental health condition that occurs in women shortly after childbirth. It is considered a psychiatric emergency due to the potential risk to the mother and to the infant.

Definition:

Postpartum psychosis is a rare and severe form of postpartum mental illness that involves a sudden onset of psychotic symptoms following childbirth. It typically occurs within the first two weeks postpartum but can develop up to 12 weeks after delivery.

Symptomatology:

Symptoms of postpartum psychosis can include:

- Delusions (false beliefs)
- Hallucinations (seeing or hearing things that are not there)
- Severe mood swings
- Disorganized thinking
- Confusion and disorientation
- Agitation and restlessness
- Insomnia
- Paranoia
- Risk of self-harm or harm to the baby

Pathophysiology:

The exact cause of postpartum psychosis is primarily clinical and involves:

- Detailed Psychiatric evaluation.

- Review of the patient's psychiatric history and family history.

- Assessment of symptoms and their onset relative to childbirth.

- Exclusion of other medical conditions that could mimic psychosis e.g. thyroid dysfunction, infections.

Prognosis:

With prompt and appropriate treatment, the progress to postpartum psychosis is generally good, with many women making a full recovery. However, there is a significant risk of recurrence in subsequent pregnancies or even outside of the postpartum period.

Complications:

If left untreated, postpartum psychosis can lead to severe complications, including:

- Suicide
- Infanticide
- Chronic psychiatric conditions
- Strained relationships and social isolation
- Impaired mother-infant bonding

Management:

Management of postpartum psychosis typically involves a combination of:

- **Hospitalization:**
  Often necessary to ensure the safety of the mother and the infant.

- **Medication:**
  - **Antipsychotics:** To manage psychotic symptoms.

- o **Mood stabilizers:** Particularly if there is an underlying bipolar disorder.

- o **Antidepressants**: May be used if depressive symptoms are prominent.

- **Electroconvulsive Therapy (ECT):**
Can be effective especially in severe cases or when rapid response is required.

- **Psychotherapy:**
Supportive therapy, cognitive- behavioral therapy (CBT) and family therapy can be beneficial.

- **Supportive Care:**
  - o Ensuring adequate sleep and nutrition.

  - o Providing emotional support and education to the patient and family.

- **Long-term Follow-up:**
Monitoring for recurrence and managing any ongoing mental health issues.

Effective management requires a multidisciplinary approach involving psychiatrists, obstetricians, pediatricians and nurses having experience in mental health, to provide comprehensive care.

CHAPTER V: IMPACT OF PARENTAL MENTAL ILLNESS ON A CHILD'S DEVELOPMENT

(A) Do Parental Mental Illness Increases the Risk to Elevate the Child's Risk of Developing Mental Illness?

The answer to this question is a big YES. Parental mental illness does elevate a child's risk of developing mental illness. This increased risk can be attributed to a combination of genetic, environmental and psychological factors. Here is a detailed look as to how these factors contribute:

Genetic Factors:

Hereditary Transmission:

Mental illness often has a genetic component, meaning children of parents with mental health disorders are at higher risk of inheriting those disorders. Conditions like depression, anxiety, bipolar disorder and schizophrenia have been shown to have well documented genetic links.

If a mother alone suffers from a mental health disorder, the child has an increased risk of developing similar issues. For example, children of a mother with depression are about three times more likely to experience depression themselves. (HealthyChildren.org) (Education Policy Institute).

If both parents are with mental disorders, the risk is substantially higher. For instance, the risk of a child developing schizophrenia is around 6% if one parent has the disorder, but it increases to 45% if both parents are affected (Verywell Mind). Similarly, for bipolar disorder, the risk is about 5% with one affected parent and rises to 40% if both parents are affected. (Depression and Bipolar Support Alliance) (Verywell Mind).

Environmental Factors:

- **Home Environment:**
  A home environment characterized by instability, high stress and lack of emotional support can contribute to the development of mental health issues in children.

- **Modeling behaviors:**
  Children may model a maladaptive behaviors and coping mechanisms of their parents, leading to the development of similar mental health issues.

- **Parental Availability:**
  Mental illness in a parent can limit their emotional availability and responsiveness, leading to attachment issues and emotional insecurity in children.

Psychological Factors:

- **Stress and Trauma:**
  Exposure to parental mental illness can be a significant source of chronic stress and trauma for children, which is a known risk factor for developing mental health disorders.

- **Emotional and Social Development:**
  As previously mentioned, difficulties in emotional regulation, social skills and self-esteem can increase vulnerability to mental health problems.

Interplay of Factors:

- **Bidirectional Influence:**

  The interaction between genetic predisposition and environmental stressors can create a feedback loop where children are not only genetically predisposed to mental health issues but are also exposed to environments that exacerbate these risks.

- **Critical Periods:**
  Certain developmental periods are more sensitive to these influences. Early childhood and adolescence are particularly critical times when exposure to parental mental illness can have a profound impact on mental health outcomes.

Evidence and Research:

- **Higher Prevalence:**
  Studies have consistently shown that children of parents with mental illness are more likely to develop mental health issues themselves. For example, children of parents with depression are more likely to experience depression and anxiety.

- **Specific Disorders:**
  The risk is not limited to the same type of mental illness. For instance, a child of a parent with depression might develop anxiety, conduct disorders or substance abuse problems.

Understanding these risks, highlight the importance of providing comprehensive support to families where a parent has a mental illness. Early identification and intervention, along with a supportive and stable environment, can help mitigate these risks and promote better mental health outcomes for children. Access to mental health care and early interventions for both parents and children can significantly reduce the risk and severity of mental health problems.

(B) Impact of Parental Mental Illness on Child's Development:

The impact of parental mental health problems on a child's development can be significant and multifaceted, affecting various domain of their growth. The adverse effects on intellectual, emotional, social and psychological development are enumerated as below.

Intellectual Development:

- **Cognitive Impairment:**
  Children may experience delays in cognitive development due to reduced parental involvement in stimulating activities, such as reading or educational play.

- **Academic Performance:**
  Lower academic achievement can occur due to inconsistent support, a chaotic home environment and frequent school absentees linked to family stress.

- **Attention and Concentration:**
  Exposure to parental mental health issues can result in difficulties with attention, focus and concentration, impacting learning and academic tasks.

Emotional Development:

- **Emotional Dysregulation:**
  Children may have difficulty managing their emotions, leading to frequent mood swings, anxiety and depressive symptoms.

- **Attachment Issues:**
  Insecure attachment patterns can develop resulting in children feeling less secure and more anxious about their relationships.

- **Sense of Security:**
  A lack of emotional stability and predictability at home can undermine a child's sense of safety and security.

Social Development:

- **Social Skills Deficits:**
  Children may struggle with developing appropriate social skills, including communication and conflict resolution, leading to difficulties in forming and maintaining friendships.

- **Social Withdrawal:**
  Increased risk of social isolation and withdrawal, as children might feel embarrassed or stigmatized by their parent's condition or lack of opportunities for social interaction.

- **Behavioral Issues:**
  Higher likelihood of exhibiting externalizing behaviors, such as aggression, defiance or delinquency which can hinder social relationships and integration.

Psychological Development:

- **Identity and Self-Esteem:**
  Parental mental health problems can affect a child's self-concept and self-esteem, leading to feelings of worthlessness or inferiority.

- **Coping Mechanisms:**
  Children may develop maladaptive coping strategies, such as substance abuse or self-harm, in response to the stress of their home environment.

- **Intergenerational Transmission:**
  There is a risk of intergenerational transmission of mental health issues, where children may develop similar mental health problems due to genetic predisposition and environmental factors.

Addressing parental mental issues through appropriate treatment and support can play a crucial role in enhancing the developmental outcome.

(C) At what age group, the child is more vulnerable to parental mental health problems??

Children are particularly vulnerable to the impact to the parental mental health problems at various stages of their development, but some periods are more critical due to the specific developmental milestones and needs associated with those ages. Here is a breakdown of these critical periods and the reasons for their heightened vulnerability:

Infancy (0 – 2 years):

- **Attachment formation:**
  This is a crucial period for forming secular attachments. Consistent responsive caregiving is essential for healthy emotional and social development. Parental mental illness can interfere with parent's ability to provide this, leading to insecure attachment patterns.

- **Brain Development:**
  Rapid brain development during infancy makes children highly sensitive to their environment, stress and loss of nurturing can negatively affect brain growth and emotional regulation.

Early Childhood (3- 6 years):

- **Emotional and Social Skills:**
  Early childhood is critical for developing basic emotional and social skills. Children learn through interaction with their parents and parental mental health issues can disrupt these interactions, leading to difficulties in emotional regulation.

- **Cognitive Development:**
  This period involves significant cognitive development, including language acquisition and basic problem-solving skills. Parental mental illness can limit stimulation and engagement, impacting cognitive growth.

Middle Childhood (7 – 12 years):

- **Self-Esteem and Competence:**
  During middle childhood, children develop self-esteem and a sense of competence through school and social activities. Parental mental illness can lead to a lack of support, guidance and stability, affecting their confidence and academic performance.

- **Understanding of Mental Illness:**
  Children start to become more aware of their parent's mental health issues, which can cause confusion, guilt and anxiety. They may also take on caregiving roles prematurely, impacting their own development.

Adolescence (13 – 18 years):

- **Identity Formation:**
  Adolescence is the critical period for identity formation and independence. Parental mental health issues can disturb this process, leading to confusion and difficulties in establishing a stable sense of self.

- **Peer Relationships:**
  Teenagers place a high value on peer relationships. Stigma and the stress of dealing with the parent's mental illness can lead to social isolation, bullying or difficulty forming healthy relationships.

- **Risk Behaviors:**
  Adolescents are more likely to engage in risk behaviors, such as substance abuse, as a way of coping with stress and instability caused by parental mental illness.

Why these ages are more vulnerable??

- **Dependency:**
  Younger children are entirely dependent on their parents for emotional and physical needs, making them particularly vulnerable to the impact of parental mental health problems.

- **Developmental Milestones:**
  Each stage has specific developmental milestones that require stable, supportive environments to achieve. Parental mental illness can disrupt the achievement of these milestones

- **Cognitive and Emotional Understanding:**
  As children grow, their understanding of their environment and their parent's behavior evolves. This awareness can lead to increased anxiety and stress, especially if they feel responsible for their parent's wellbeing.

Understanding these vulnerabilities, underscores the importance of providing targeted support and interventions at different developmental stages to help children cope with and overcome the challenges posed by parental mental health problems.

(D) How to reduce the chances of child developing mental issues, if one or both parents are suffering from mental health disorders??

Reducing the chances of child developing mental health issues when parents suffer from the same, involves addressing both genetic predispositions and environmental factors. Here are systemic steps to mitigate the risks.

Provide a Supportive Environment:

- **Consistent Routines:**
  Establishing and maintaining daily routines can provide children with a sense of stability and security.

- **Safe and Nurturing Home:**
  Ensure that the home environment is safe, nurturing and free from abuse or neglect. This includes addressing any domestic violence or substance abuse issues.

- **Open Communication:**
  Encourage open and honest communication about feelings and experiences, fostering a supportive and understanding atmosphere. (Education Policy Institute) (MDPI).

Mental Health Support for Parents:

- **Professional Treatment:**
  Parents should seek appropriate treatment for their mental health issues, such as therapy, medication or both. Proper management of their conditions can significantly reduce the negative impact on their children (HeathyChildren.org).

- **Parenting Programs:**
  Engage in parenting programs designed to support parents with mental health issues, helping them develop effective parenting strategies and coping mechanisms (MDPI).

Early Intervention and Monitoring:

- **Regular Check-ups:**
  Children should have regular mental health check-ups to monitor for early signs of mental health issues.

- **Early Intervention Services:**
  If any issues are detected, early intervention services can provide support to address these problems before they escalate (Education Policy Institute) (Verywell Mind).

Promote Healthy Lifestyle Choices:

- **Nutrition and Exercise:**
  Encourage a balanced diet and regular physical activity, which can improve overall mental health and reduce stress and anxiety (Verywell Mind).

- **Adequate Sleep:**
  Ensure that children get sufficient sleep, as poor sleep can contribute to the onset of mental health issues (Verywell Mind).

Educational Support:

- **School Resources:**
  Utilize school resources such as counseling services, special education programs and after-school activities to support children's emotional and educational needs.

- **Parental Involvement:**
  Stay involved in the child's education by regularly communicating with teachers and school counselors about any concerns or needs. (Education Policy Institute).

Stress Management Techniques:

- **Mindfulness and Relaxation:**
  Teach children mindfulness, relaxation techniques and coping strategies to manage stress and anxiety effectively.

- **Therapeutic Activities:**
  Encourage activities that promote mental wellbeing such as art, music and play therapy (Verywell Mind).

Professional Therapy for Children:

- **Individual Therapy:**
  Consider individual therapy for children to help them process their experiences and develop healthy coping mechanisms.

- **Family Therapy:**
  Engage in family therapy to address and resolve family dynamics that may contribute to mental health issues. (MDPI).

Implementing these strategies can help mitigate the impact of parental mental health disorders on children, promoting healthier development and reducing the likelihood of children developing similar issues.

CHATER VI: MENTAL HEALTH IN MENOPAUSE

"Embrace the change,

it's a beginning of a new, vibrant chapter."

(A) Definition of Menopause:

- Menopause is defined by Stedman as permanent cessation of menses. An awareness of menopause can be traced from ancient Greeks. In fact, the word menopause is derived from the Greek word meno meaning month and refers to menstrual cycle, while pause meaning to cease or to stop. In other words, menopause literally means cessation of monthly cycles.

- **The World Health Organization (WHO)** has defined natural menopause as the permanent cessation of menses resulting from loss of ovarian follicular activity. Menopause marks the end of reproductive life and natural menopause is the retrospective clinical diagnosis which occurs after 12 consecutive months of amenorrhoea, for which no other pathological cause can be established.

- The menopausal transition is the time before the final menopausal period **(FMP)** and is associated with irregular cycles, hormonal instability and symptoms.

Pathophysiology of Menopause Transition:

- **Biology of ovarian aging:**

In the human ovary, there is a continuous and progressive decline in the number of follicles from foetal life onwards. From several million follicles present at birth, less than a thousand remain at menopause. The loss cannot be accounted for by ovulation alone. Because the reproductive span of 30-35 years in a woman can only account for a loss of 350-450 ovarian follicles through ovulation. Their disappearance is also related to a loss of oocytes and surrounding granulosa and theca cells of the ovarian follicles that occur continuously through a process of follicular atresia. In every cycle, from a recruited pool of growing follicles, only one dominant follicle is selected, the rest undergoing atresia. It is clear from several studies **(Block 1952, Gougeon 1984, Gosden 1985, Richardson et al 1987)** that serum gonadotropins mainly follicular stimulating hormone (FSH) are responsible for accelerating the pace of follicular atresia leading to the depletion of stock and subsequent menopause.

- **Menopause Markers (Hormonal Changes during menopause transition):**

The transition from the ovulatory cycles to the menopausal state is usually not an instantaneous event. Rather it is a series of hormonal clinical alterations that reflect declining ovarian function. Menopause is diagnosed retrospectively by history. Markers for diagnosis of menopause are preferably restricted for use in special situations and for fertility issues.

- **FSH** > 10 IU/L is indicative of declining ovarian function.

- **FSH** > 20 IU/L is diagnostic of ovarian failure in the perimenopausal age group with vasomotor symptoms (VMS) even in the absence of complete cessation of menses.

- **FSH** > 40 IU/L done 2 months apart is diagnostic of menopause.

- **FSH** rise precedes the LH rise.

- **FSH** is a diagnostic marker of ovarian failure while **LH** is not.

- **LH** measurement is not necessary to make a diagnosis of menopause.

- 1 - 3 years after menopause, serum **LH** rises by **3 folds** while **FSH** by **10 - 20 folds.** Rise in serum **LH** level is less pronounced than serum **FSH** level because **LH** has a shorter half-life period and has no specific negative peptide. **(FSH has a specific negative feedback peptide called Inhibin.)**

- **Postmenopausal serum estradiol level falls and it is < 20 pg/ml at menopause.** (Premenopausal level of serum estradiol varies from 40 -400 pg/ml).

- **AMH** and **Inhibin** levels are low or undetectable at menopause. Inhibin is a polypeptide that is secreted by granulosa cells, it has both paracrine and endocrine functions. At the central level inhibin exerts a negative feedback effect and reduces the pituitary secretion of FSH. At the ovarian level its paracrine function is to prevent folliculogenesis of other follicles. An increasing level of serum FSH during early follicular phase and a decline in circulating levels of inhibin and estradiol are the first indications of age-related acceleration of follicular depletion. Serum inhibin during the early follicular phase showed a significant decline in women of 45-49 years of age as compared to those aged below 45 years **(McLachlan et.al. 1987-88).**

➢ On transvaginal ultrasound the antral follicular count is low and ovarian volume is also reduced.

• **Estrogen/Testosterone Shift in Menopausal Women and other related factors:**

During menopause, significant hormonal changes occur in women's body, particularly involving estrogen and testosterone. This Estrogen/Testosterone shift has profound effect on both physical and mental health.

o **Estrogen Decline:** Normal serum estradiol level in women in reproductive age group is 40 – 400 pg/ml depending up on the stage of menstrual cycle. Estrogen is a key hormone in female sexual health. It is responsible for maintaining the health of vaginal tissues, promoting lubrication and supporting the overall sexual response cycle. Estradiol level in postmenopausal women is below 20 pg/ml. After menopause, ovaries no longer produce estrogen. Instead, in small amounts it is produced in a number of extra-gonadal sites such as kidney, adipose tissue, skin and brain. Unlike ovarian synthesized estrogen, which is released into the blood stream, estrogen synthesized within these extra-gonadal sites mostly acts locally at the site of synthesis and functions as a paracrine and/or intracrine factor to maintain important tissue specific functions.

- o **Impact on Body:**

  - ✓ **Vasomotor Symptoms:** The decline in estrogen is responsible for common menopausal symptoms such as hot flashes and night sweats.

  - ✓ **Bone Health:** Reduced estrogen levels lead to decreased bone density, increasing the risk of osteoporosis.

  - ✓ **Cardiovascular Health:** Estrogen has protective effects on the heart and blood vessels; its decline can lead to an increased risk of cardiovascular diseases.
  - ✓ **Mental Health:** Estrogen influence neurotransmitter systems that regulate mood and cognitive functions. Its decrease can lead to symptoms such as depression, anxiety and cognitive decline.

- o **Relative Increase in Testosterone:** While testosterone levels also decline during menopause, the decrease is more gradual compared to estrogen. As a result, there is a relative increase in androgen-to-estrogen ratio. This shift can lead to noticeable changes in a woman's body.

- o **Effect of the Estrogen / Testosterone Shift:**
  - ✓ **Androgenic Symptoms:** The relative increase in testosterone can cause symptoms such as thinning scalp hair, increased facial hairs and a deeper voice.

- ✓ **Libido Changes:** Testosterone plays a role in sexual desire, and the hormonal shift during menopause can lead to changes in libido, with some women experiencing a decrease and others in increase in sexual interest.

  - ✓ **Muscle Mass:** Testosterone helps maintain muscle mass, so while overall muscle mass may decline with aging, the relative increase in testosterone can help in preserving it to some extent

- o **Overall Impact:**
  The estrogen/testosterone shift during menopause contribute to a range of physical and mental health changes. The decline in estrogen is primarily responsible for the more commonly recognised symptoms of menopause, such as hot flashes, mood swings and increased risk of osteoporosis and cardiovascular issues. Meanwhile the relative increase in sexual function, body function, and the emergence of androgenic symptoms.

- **Changes in cycle length and menstrual bleeding:** Women aged 18-24 years have an average follicular phase length of 15 ± 2 days, but those aged 40 -44 years have an average length of $10 + 2$ days, which tends to shorten the menstrual cycle. Thus, menstrual cycle length may shorten before it lengthens as women progress through the transition. **(Trealar et. al. 1967)**

One hallmark of the menopause transition is a change in bleeding pattern, **Van Voorhis and et. al.** has studied hormonal pattern and menstrual bleeding pattern in a large sub cohort of the **SWAN** participants aged 42-52 years. They found that 20% of all cycles during the time were an ovulatory. They also noted that short cycle lengths (<21 days) were common early in menopause transition whereas long cycle intervals (> 36 days) were associated with late menopause transition.

(B) Age at Menopause:

- The menopause transition most often begins between ages 45 and 55 years. The average age at menopause of an Indian woman is 46.2 years, much less than western woman (51 years).

- From available Indian data it is hypothesized that an early age at menopause in Indian women (46.2 years) predisposes them to chronic health disorders a decade earlier than the Caucasians having late age at menopause (51 years).

- It is reported that osteoporotic fractures occur 10-20 years earlier in Indians as compared to Caucasians.

- The first myocardial infarction (MI) attack occurs in 4.4% of Asian women at a younger age than in European women.

- In India, type II diabetes occurs a decade earlier than the Caucasians.

- Breast cancer is the most common cancer in Indian women and the incidence peaks before the age of 50 years.

As the women approach their mid-forties, many women find themselves looking for signs of menopause and trying to figure out when it will begin for them. Most women reach menopause between the ages of 45 and 55 years. But as every woman is unique, age at menopause may also differ due to underlying conditions.

- **Genetic factors:**
  Research has conclusively shown that there is a strong link between menopause and genetics. There are approximately 50% chances that a woman will become menopausal at the same age as her mother or within a few years of that age. However, this may not always be the case.

- **Ethnicity:**
  Studies have conclusively revealed that the average menopausal age for Caucasian women in the UK and USA is around 51 years, while in Indians it is 46.2 yrs. The reason for these variations is that women of different ethnicities often have different levels of estrogenic activity.

- **Smoking**:
  Smoking has been found to be the number one modifiable lifestyle factor relating to early menopause. Polycyclic aromatic hydrocarbons found in cigarette smoke are toxic to ovarian follicles. These chemicals can cause premature loss of follicles leading to early onset of menopause.
  Smoking can lead to faster breakdown of oestrogen in the liver which in turn results in an earlier decline in oestrogen level.

- **Body Mass Index (BMI):**
  A study conducted by Australian University has shown that women who are underweight or have a low BMI are more likely to enter menopause early, while women who are overweight or have high BMI

are more likely to experience a late menopause. This is due to the fact that oestrogen is stored in fat cells.

- **Parity**:
Nulliparous women may experience an earlier menopause while multiparty or a late first pregnancy may result in a later onset.

- **Other factors include:**
Women with bilateral oophorectomy, exposure to radiotherapy or chemotherapy in premenopausal age experience early induced menopause.

- Use of oral contraceptives may delay the onset.

Is there a menopause age calculator?

All factors discussed above could help women to determine the appropriate age at menopause but there is no definite test to predict it. In a nutshell AMH levels indicate the number of follicles present in the ovaries and unlike FSH levels, AMH levels do not fluctuate with phases in menstrual cycles, which means that they can be used to determine the extent of ovarian reserve and thereby the approximate age at which menopause will occur.

Terminologies in relation to menopause:

- **Natural Menopause:**
  It is recognised to have occurred after 12 months of amenorrhoea for which there are no obvious pathological causes.

- **Premenopause:**
  It is often used to refer to the entire reproductive period up to the final menstrual period (FMP).

- **Perimenopause:**
  It is the period immediately before 2 - 3 years and 1 year after FMP. It may last up to 3 - 5 yrs. The characteristics are:
  - Increasing serum FSH levels
  - Significantly reduced fertility
  - Erratic menstrual periods
  - Onset of menstrual symptoms

  (The term is used interchangeably with menopause transition.)

- **Climacteric:**
  It is interchangeably used with perimenopause and menopause transition. When associated with symptoms, it is called climacteric syndrome.

- **Postmenopause:**
  It is the span of life dating from the final menstrual period onwards regardless of whether the menopause was spontaneous or iatrogenic.

- **Premature Ovarian Insufficiency (POI):**
  Premature ovarian Insufficiency has replaced the term premature menopause. POI is described as amenorrhoea due to loss of ovarian function before the age of 40 years. It is a state of female

hypergonadotrophic hypogonadism. Its incidence is 1%. It can manifest as primary amenorrhoea with onset before menarche or secondary amenorrhoea with onset after the establishment of natural menses. Criteria for diagnosis of POI as per *European Society of Human Reproduction and Embryology (ESHRE 2015) is 'Elevated FSH levels > 25 IU/L on two occasions > 4 weeks apart'*.

- **Early Menopause**:
  It is the time span between the spontaneous or iatrogenic menopause occurring between 40 years of age and the accepted typical age of menopause for a given population (between 40 and 46.2 years in Indian population). Incidence is 5%.

- **Delayed Menopause:**
  It is not well defined but may be important in terms of increased problems associated with hyperestrogenism. It is two SDs above from the natural average age of menopause in a given population. In India, we may consider it to be 54 years or more.

- **Postmenopausal Bleeding (PMB):**
  It is the bleeding which occurs 12 months after the last menstrual period. However, it is recommended that any vaginal bleeding that occurs 6 months after the last menstrual period should be investigated.

- **Induced Menopause/Surgical Menopause**:
  It is the cessation of menses due to bilateral oophorectomy or iatrogenic ablation of ovarian function or hysterectomy.

(C) Symptoms of Menopause:

- About 20% of women have no symptoms at all, while 60% have mild to moderate symptoms. The remaining 20% have severe symptoms that interfere with their daily life.

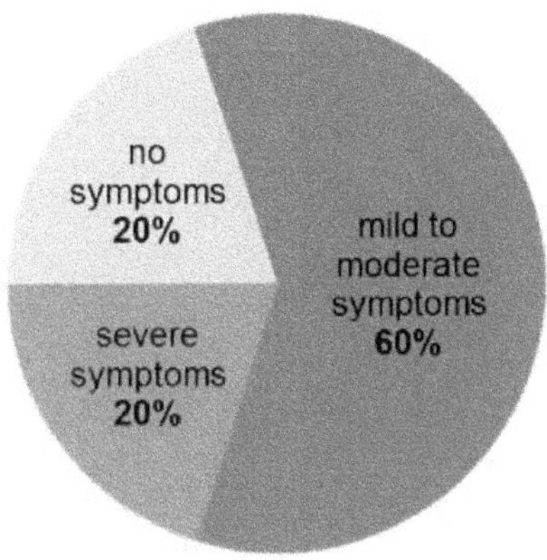

- Menopausal symptoms can be influenced by different factors, for example, your stage of life and general health and wellbeing.

- The biology and symptomatology of menopause is blurred due to its relationship to the underlying aging process.

- Vasomotor, urogenital symptoms and irregular menstrual periods are typically linked with serum oestrogen levels.

- Long term effects on bone and heart have been related to oestrogen deficiency.

- Many other symptoms like muscle and joint pain, vertigo, mood changes, depression, insomnia, nervousness have been associated with menopause but are not necessarily due to decrease in oestrogen levels.

- Many symptoms start during perimenopause and can continue into postmenopause. Australian studies show that some women experience symptoms like hot flashes and night sweats well into their 60s.

Physical Symptoms:

Physical symptoms may include:

- Irregular periods
- Hot flashes
- Night sweats
- Sleep problems
- Sore breasts
- Itchy, crawly or dry skin
- Exhaustion and fatigue
- Dry vagina
- Loss of sex drive (libido)
- Headaches or migraine
- Aches and pains
- Bloating
- Urinary problems
- Weight gains due to androgen-oestrogen ratio shift and low BMR.

Emotional symptoms may include:

- Feeling irritable or frustrated
- Feeling anxious
- Difficulty in concentrating
- Forgetfulness
- Mood swings

Symptoms and Disorders in Relation to Age and Menopause:

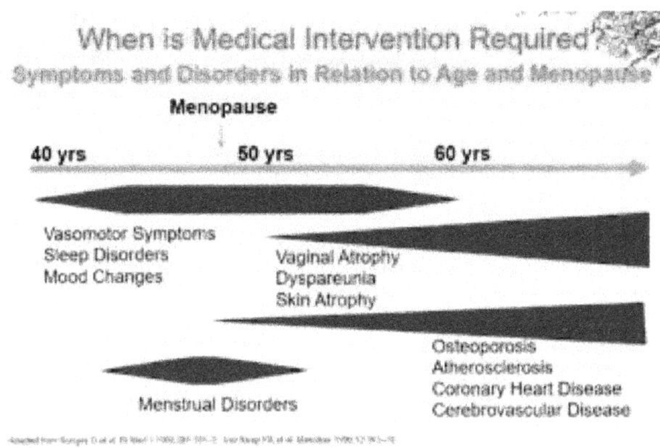

Source: Bungay G, et al. Br Med J 1980; 281: 181 - 3;

Van Keep PA, et al. Maturities 1990; 12:163-70.

> *The immediate symptoms of menopause transition are irregular periods, hot flashes, night sweats, sleep and mood disturbances, joint and muscle pain, vaginal dryness and low sexual desire which generally resolve over a while in mild cases.*

> *Genitourinary symptoms appear in the early postmenopausal period and may worsen over some time if not treated.*

> *The long-term consequences of menopause affect bone and cardiovascular health which worsen with aging.*

(D) Mental Health in Menopause:

Menopause, a natural biological process that marks the end of a woman's menstrual cycles, often brings significant hormonal changes. These changes can lead to various physical and mental health issues. One of the critical aspects of menopause is the decline in the levels of estrogen and progesterone, which can significantly affect mental health. Here is a closer look at how hormonal imbalances during menopause can impact mental health.

Common Mental Health Issues during Menopause:

- **Depression:**
    - Decrease estrogen levels can affect serotonin production, a neurotransmitter linked to mood regulation. This can increase the risk of depression.

    - Women with a history of depression or premenstrual syndrome (PMS) are particularly more susceptible.

- **Anxiety:**
    - Hormonal fluctuations can trigger anxiety, manifesting as general anxiety, panic attacks or increased nervousness.

    - Estrogen helps regulate the stress response, and its decline can lead to heightened anxiety levels.

- **Mood Swings:**
  - o Rapid changes in hormone levels can lead to unpredictable mood swings, similar to those experienced during PMS, but often more intense.

  - o These mood swings can contribute to irritability, frustration and emotional instability.

- **Memory Problems and Cognitive Decline:**
  - o Some women experience "brain fog", which includes difficulties with concentration, memory and cognitive functions.

  - o Estrogen has a protective effect on the brain, and its reduction can lead to cognitive issues.

- **Sleep Disturbances:**
  - o Menopause often brings sleep problems, such as insomnia or disturbed sleep due to night sweats and hot flushes.

  - o Poor sleep quality can exacerbate mental health issues like depression and anxiety.

Mechanisms behind Hormonal Impact:

What Role Neurotransmitters Play in our Body in General?

Neurotransmitters play a crucial role in the communication between neurons in the nervous system. They are chemical messengers that transmit signals across synapses, the gaps between neurons, to ensure proper functioning of the brain and the nervous system. Here is a general review of their role:

- **Signal Transmission:**
  Neurotransmitters are released from the axon terminals of a neuron in response to an electrical signal. (Action potential). They cross the synaptic cleft and bind to receptors on the surface of the target neuron, muscle cells or gland which triggers a response in the receiving cell.

- **Regulation of Mood and Emotion:**
  Neurotransmitters such as serotonin and dopamine are crucial for mood regulation, emotional responses and feelings of pleasure and reward. Imbalances in these neurotransmitters are linked to conditions like depression and anxiety.

- **Cognitive Functions:**
  Acetylcholine and glutamate are essential for cognitive functions, including memory, learning and attention. They facilitate communication in areas of the brain involved in the processes.

- **Control of Movement:**
  Dopamine and acetylcholine are involved in regulation of motor control. Dopamine, for example, plays a significant role in the coordination of

movements and is notably affected in Parkinson's disease.

- **Autonomic Functions:**
Neurotransmitters like norepinephrine and acetylcholine are involved in the autonomic nervous system, regulating involuntary functions such as heart rate, digestion, respiratory rate and blood pressure.

- **Pain Perception:**
Endorphins and encephalin are neurotransmitters that modulate pain perception and are part of body's natural pain relief system.

Neurotransmitters are essential for maintaining the body's homeostasis and over being by ensuring effective communication within the nervous system. Disruptions in neurotransmitter systems can lead to various neurological and psychiatric disorders, highlighting their importance in maintaining mental and physical health.

(E) Impact of Estrogen Deficiency on Neurotransmitters:

- **Effect on Serotonin:**
  - **Synthesis:**
    - ✓ Estrogen increases the expression of tryptophan hydroxylase, the enzyme responsible for serotonin synthesis.

    - ✓ With reduced estrogen, serotonin production declines.

  - **Metabolism:**
    - ✓ Estrogen influences the breakdown of serotonin by affecting the activity of monoamine oxidase (MAO), and enzyme that degrade serotonin.

    - ✓ Lower estrogen level results in increased MAO activity, leading to decreased serotonin availability.

  - **Receptor Function:**
    - ✓ Estrogen modulates the sensitivity and density of serotonin receptors.

    - ✓ Deficiency can lead to reduced receptor sensitivity, impairing serotonin signaling.

- **Effect on Dopamine:**
  - **Synthesis:**
    - ✓ Estrogen enhances the activity of tyrosine hydroxylase, the enzyme involved in dopamine synthesis.

- ✓ Reduced estrogen level leads to decreased dopamine production.

  - o **Metabolism:**
    - ✓ Estrogen affects the activity of enzymes like catechol-O-methyl transferase (COMT) that degreed dopamine.

    - ✓ Lower estrogen levels result in faster dopamine degradation, reducing its availability.

  - o **Receptor Function:**
    - ✓ Estrogen influences dopamine receptor density and function particularly D2 receptors.

    - ✓ Estrogen deficiency can decrease receptor density, impairing dopamine signaling.

- **Effect on Noradrenaline:**
  - o **Synthesis:**
    - ✓ Estrogen stimulates the synthesis of norepinephrine by enhancing the activity of enzymes involved in its production.

    - ✓ Lower estrogen levels can lead to reduced norepinephrine synthesis.

  - o **Metabolism:**
    - ✓ Estrogen modulates the breakdown of norepinephrine by affecting the activity of enzymes such as MAO.

    - ✓ With decreased estrogen levels, increased enzyme activity leads to lower norepinephrine levels.

- o **Receptor Function:**
  - ✓ Estrogen affects the sensitivity and density of norepinephrine receptors.

  - ✓ Deficiency can lead to reduced receptor sensitivity and altered norepinephrine signaling.

Role of Serotonin, Dopamine and Norepinephrine in Mood Stability and Cognitive Function:

- **Mood Stability:**
  - o **Serotonin:**
    - ✓ High levels of serotonin are associated with improved mood and emotional stability.

    - ✓ Reduced Serotonin due to estrogen deficiency can lead to mood swings, depression and anxiety.

  - o **Dopamine:**
    - ✓ Dopamine is crucial for pleasure, reward and motivation.

    - ✓ Decreased Dopamine levels can contribute to anhedonia (inability to experience joy or pleasure), low motivation and depression.

  - o **Norepinephrine:**
    - ✓ Norepinephrine is involved in the body's stress response and alertness.

    - ✓ Reduced levels can lead to fatigue, decreased concentration and mood instability.

- **Cognitive Function:**
  - **Serotonin:**
    - ✓ Serotonin influences cognitive functions such as memory and learning.

    - ✓ Reduced Serotonin levels can impair these functions, contributing to "brain fog" and memory problems.

  - **Dopamine:**
    - ✓ Dopamine is essential for executive functions, including working memory, attention and problem-solving.

    - ✓ Lower Dopamine levels can impair these cognitive processes, affecting overall cognitive performance.

  - **Norepinephrine:**
    - ✓ Norepinephrine enhances attention, arousal and reaction time.

    - ✓ Deficiency can lead to difficulties with attention and slower cognitive processing.

Estrogen deficiency during menopause disrupts the synthesis, metabolism and receptor function of key neurotransmitters such as serotonin, dopamine and norepinephrine. These disruptions contribute to mood instability and cognitive decline. Understanding these mechanisms, highlights the importance of addressing estrogen deficiency to maintain mental and cognitive health during menopause.

(F) Role of Progesterone in Regulating Anxiety:

Progesterone plays a significant role in regulating anxiety by interacting with gamma-aminobutyric acid (GABA) receptors in the brain. The deficiency of progesterone during menopause can influence this effect, leading to increased anxiety and other mood disturbances. Here is a systematic enumeration.

- **Interaction with GABA receptors:**
  - **GABA Receptors:**
  GABA is the primary inhibitory transmitter in the brain, which helps to reduce neuronal excitability and promote a calming effect.

  GABA receptors are the sites where GABA binds to exert its inhibitory effects.
  - **Progesterone Metabolites:**
  Progesterone is metabolized into allopregnanolone, a neuroactive steroid.

  Allopregnanolone binds to GABA_A receptors, enhancing their inhibitory effects.

  - **Enhancing GABAergic Activity:**
  When allopregnanolone binds to GABA_A receptors, it increases the receptors response to GABA.

  This potentiation leads to enhanced inhibitory signaling, promoting relaxation and reducing anxiety.

- **Effects on the Brain:**
  - **Calming Effect:**
    By enhancing GABAergic activity, allopregnanolone helps to calm neuronal activity, reducing symptoms of anxiety and promoting a sense of wellbeing.

  - **Mood Stabilization:**
    Progesterone's metabolites help stabilize mood by counteracting the excitatory neurotransmitter effects in the brain, contributing to emotional stability.

  - **Sleep Regulation:**
    The interaction with $GABA\_A$ receptors also helps to regulate sleep, promoting better sleep quality and reducing insomnia.

Influence of Progesterone Deficiency during Menopause:

- **Decreased GABAergic Activity:**
  - **Lower Allopregnanolone Levels:**
    During menopause, progesterone levels drop, leading to reduced production of allopregnanolone.

  - **Reduced GABA Potentiation:**
    With less allopregnanolone available to enhance $GABA\_A$ receptor function, GABAergic inhibitory efforts are diminished.

  - **Increased Neural Excitability:**
    The reduction in inhibitory signaling leads to increased neural excitability, contributing to heightened anxiety.

- **Increased Anxiety:**
  - o **Reduced Calming Effects:**
    The diminished interaction with GABA_A receptors means the brain's natural calming mechanisms are less effective.

  - o **Heightened Stress Response:**
    The lack of adequate GABAergic activity can lead to an overactive stress response, making individuals more susceptible to anxiety and panic attacks.

- **Mood Instability:**
  - o **Emotional Variability:**
    The stabilizing effect of progesterone on mood is lost, leading to greater emotional variability and mood swings.

  - o **Increased Irritability:**
    Reduced calming effects contribute to irritability and emotional sensitivity.

- **Sleep Disturbances:**
  - o **Insomnia:**
    Decreased GABAergic activity can disturb sleep patterns, leading to insomnia and poor sleep quality.

  - o **Poor Sleep Quality:**
    Inadequate sleep further exacerbates anxiety and disturbances, creating a vicious cycle.

Progesterone helps to regulate anxiety through its metabolite allopregnanolone, which enhances the inhibitory effects of GABA by interacting with GABA_A receptors. This interaction promotes a calming effect on the brain, reduces anxiety and stabilizes mood. During menopause, progesterone deficiency leads to decreased allopregnanolone levels, reducing GABAergic activity. This deficiency increases neural excitability and sleep disturbances. Understanding these mechanisms underscores the importance of managing progesterone levels to maintain mental health during menopause.

Influence of Deficiency of Hormones other than Estrogen and Progesterone:

In addition to estrogen and progesterone, other hormone deficiencies during menopause, such as those of testosterone, (DHEA), can significantly influence mental health problems. Here is a systemic enumeration.

Testosterone Deficiency:

- **Role in Mental Health:**
  - **Mood Regulation:**
    Testosterone contributes to mood regulation and a sense of wellbeing.

  - **Libido:**
    It plays a role in maintaining sexual desire, which can affect overall quality of life and mental health.

  - **Cognitive Function:**
    Testosterone is involved in cognitive functions, including memory, attention and spatial abilities.

- **Effect of Deficiency:**
  - **Depression:**
    Lower testosterone levels can contribute to feelings of depression and low mood.

  - **Anxiety:**
    Some women may experience increased anxiety and irritability.

  - **Cognitive Decline:**
    Deficiency may lead to memory problems and difficulty with concentration.

Thyroid Hormone Deficiency:

- **Role in Mental Health:**
  - o **Metabolism Regulation**
    Thyroid hormones (T3 and T4) are crucial for regulating metabolism, energy levels and overall brain function.

  - o **Mood Stability:**
    Adequate thyroid function support mood stability and cognitive health.

- **Effect of Deficiency (Hypothyroidism):**
  - o **Depression:**
    Hypothyroidism is often associated with symptoms of depression, including low energy, sadness and lethargy.

  - o **Anxiety:**
    Some individuals may experience increased anxiety and nervousness.

  - o **Cognitive Impairment:**
    Deficiency can lead to cognitive symptoms such as memory problems, difficulty concentrating and slowed thinking.

Dehydroepiandrosterone Deficiency:

- **Role in Mental Health:**
  - o **Precursor to other hormones:**
    DHEA is a precursor to estrogen and progesterone, contributing to their production.

o **Stress Response:**
  DHEA helps to modulate the body's stress response and anti-stress effects.

- **Effects of Deficiency:**
  o **Mood Disorders:**
    Low levels of DHEA are associated with mood disorders, including depression and anxiety.

  o **Cognitive Function:**
    DHEA deficiency may contribute to cognitive decline, affecting memory and executive functions.

Cortisol Dysregulation:

- **Role in Mental Health:**
  o **Stress Hormone:**
    Cortisol is the primary stress hormone, playing a key role in the body's response to stress.

  o **Mood and Energy:**
    Proper cortisol levels are important for maintaining energy levels and emotional stability.

- **Effects of Dysregulation:**
  o **Increased Anxiety:**
    Dysregulated cortisol levels can lead to chronic stress and anxiety.

  o **Depression:**
    Both elevated and insufficient cortisol levels are associated with depression.

- o **Sleep Disturbances:**
  Cortisol dysregulation can disrupt sleep patterns, leading to insomnia and poor sleep quality.

Insulin and Glucose Metabolism:

- **Role in Mental Health:**
  - o **Energy Regulation:**
    Insulin is crucial for regulating blood glucose levels and providing energy to the brain.

  - o **Mood and Cognitive Function:**
    Stable glucose levels are important for mood stability and cognitive function.

- **Effects of Dysregulation:**
  - o **Mood Swings:**
    Insulin resistance and fluctuations in blood glucose levels can lead to mood swings and irritability.

  - o **Cognitive Impairment:**
    Poor glucose regulation can contribute to cognitive problems, including memory issues and difficulty in concentrating.

Apart from estrogen and progesterone, deficiencies in testosterone, thyroid hormones, DHEA, cortisol and insulin dysregulation can significantly influence mental health during menopause. These hormonal changes can lead to a variety of mental health issues, including depression, anxiety, mood swings and cognitive decline. Understanding these influences is crucial for developing comprehensive treatment strategies to support women's mental health during menopause.

(G) How to Cope with Physical and Hormonal Changes during Menopause?

Coping with physical and hormonal changes during menopause can be challenging, but several strategies can help manage symptoms and improve overall wellbeing. Here is a systematic approach:

Healthy Lifestyle:

Lifestyle modifications can play a crucial role in improving mental health in postmenopausal women. As women transition through menopause, the physical and hormonal changes they experience can significantly impact their mental well-being. Adopting a healthy lifestyle can help mitigate these effects and promote overall mental health. Here are some lifestyle modifications that can be beneficial.

1. **Regular Physical Activity:**
   - **Exercise Benefits:**
     Engaging in regular physical activities can reduce symptoms of depression, anxiety and stress, which are common during menopause. Exercise boots the production of endorphins, the body's natural mood elevators, and help regulate sleep patterns.

   - **Types of Exercise:**
     Activities like walking, jogging, swimming, yoga and strength training can be particularly effective. Even moderate exercise, such as daily brisk walking, can make a significant difference.

2. **Healthy Diet:**
   - **Nutrient-rich foods:**
     A balanced diet rich in fruits, vegetables, whole grains, lean proteins and healthy fats can support

mental health. Omega-3 fatty acids can support mental health. Omega-3 fatty acids found in fish and flaxseeds, are known to improve mood and cognitive function.

- **Mindful Eating:**
Reducing the intake of processed foods, sugar and caffeine can help stabilize mood and energy levels. Additionally maintaining a healthy weight through mindful eating can reduce the risk of developing conditions like diabetes and heart disease, which are linked to depression.

3. **Adequate Sleep:**
   - **Sleep Hygiene:**
   The National Institute for Health (NIH) says adults need 7-8 hrs of sleep each night to stay in good mental and physical health. Poor sleep is a common issue during menopause and can exacerbate mental health problems. Establishing a regular sleep routine, creating a relaxing bedtime environment, and avoiding stimulants like caffeine, electronic media such as smart mobile, TV before bed can improve sleep.

   - **Sleep Support:**
   Practices such as mindfulness, meditation and relaxation exercises can also aid in achieving better sleep.

4. **Stress Management:**
   - **Mindfulness and Meditation:**
   Techniques such as mindfulness, meditation and deep breathing exercises can help reduce stress and anxiety, improving mental clarity and emotional stability.

- **Relaxation Activities:**
  Engaging in activities like reading, gardening or hobbies that promote relaxation can also contribute to lower stress levels.

5. **Social Connections:**
   - **Support Networks:**
     Maintaining strong social connections is essential for mental health. Regular interaction with family; friends, or support groups can provide emotional support and reduce feelings of isolation, which are common during postmenopause.

   - **Community Engagement:**
     Participating in community activities or volunteer work can also enhance a sense of purpose and well-being.

6. **Mental Health Support:**
   - **Counseling and Therapy:**
     Professional counseling or therapy can be very beneficial in managing the emotional changes that accompany menopause. Cognitive Behavior therapy (CBT) is particularly effective in addressing anxiety and depression.

   - **Mind-Body Practices:**
     Practices like yoga and tai chi combine physical activity with mindfulness, which can help in reducing anxiety and improving overall mental health.

7. **Avoiding Harmful Habits:**
   - **Limiting Alcohol and Smoking:**
     Reducing or avoiding alcohol consumption and smoking is important, as these habits can

negatively impact mood, increase anxiety and interfere with sleep.

8. **Routine Health Check-Ups:**
   - **Regular Monitoring:**
     Regular health check-ups can help in early detection and management of health issues that can impact mental health, such as thyroid problems or cardiovascular conditions.

In conclusion, lifestyle modifications offer a natural and holistic approach to improving mental health in postmenopausal women. By incorporating regular physical activity, a balanced diet, stress management techniques and maintaining strong social connections, women can enhance their emotional well-being and navigate the challenges of menopause with greater resilience and positivity.

Empty Nest Syndrome:

Empty nest syndrome refers to the feelings of sadness, loss and emotional distress that parents may experience when their children leave home for the first time, such as going to college or for joining job or to live independently. This transition can be particularly challenging because it marks a significant change in daily routines and family dynamics.

- **Emotional Impact:**
  - ✓ **Sadness and Loneliness:**
    Parents often feel a profound sense of sadness and loneliness when the house becomes quitter and daily interactions with their children decrease.

  - ✓ **Loss of Purpose:**
    Many parents derive a strong sense of identity and purpose from their role as caregivers. When children leave, they might struggle with a sense of lost purpose.

- **Adjustment of Challenges:**
  - ✓ **Routine Changes:**
    The daily routines and activities that revolved around the children such as school events, meals and household tasks; change dramatically.

  - ✓ **Relationship Shifts:**
    The dynamics within the family and marital relationship can shift, requiring adjustments and re-evaluation roles and interactions.

- **Positive Opportunities:**
  - ✓ **Personal Growth:**
    This period can also be an opportunity for personal growth, allowing parents to rediscover individual interests and passions that may have set aside.

✓ **Marital Renewal:**
Couples can use this time to reconnect and strengthen their relationships without the focus on parenting responsibilities.

Coping with Empty Nest Syndrome:

Coping with empty nest syndrome and redefining personal identity involves several strategies:

o **Acknowledge Your Feelings:**
  ✓ **Recognize Emotions:**
  Accept that the feelings of sadness, loss or loneliness are normal and a routine happening for every parents.

  ✓ **Validate Yourself:**
  Understand that it's okay to grieve the change in your family dynamics.

o **Stay Connected:**
  ✓ **Maintain Relationships:**
  Keep in regular contact with your children through calls, massages and visits.

  ✓ **Strengthen Social Network:**
  Foster relationships with friends, neighbours and extended family.

o **Focus on Your Partner:**
  ✓ **Rekindle Romance:**
  Spend quality time with your partner, rediscover shared interests and create new memories.

✓ **Communicate:**
Discuss feelings and expectations openly to strengthen your bond.

o **Set New Goals:**
✓ **Personal Goals:**
Identify and peruse personal aspirations or interests you may have set aside.

✓ **Professional Goals:**
Consider furthering your career, starting a new job or engaging in volunteer work.

o **Create a New Routine:**
✓ **Daily Structure:**
Develop a daily routine that includes hobbies, social activities and personal time.

✓ **Physical Activity:**
Incorporate regular exercise to boost mood and energy levels.

o **Seek Support:**
✓ **Support Groups:**
Join groups for empty nesters to share experiences and gain support.

✓ **Therapy:**
Seek counselling if feelings of sadness or anxiety become overwhelming.

Redefine Personal Identity:

o **Self-Reflection:**
  - ✓ **Assess Interest:**
    Reflect on your interests, values and passions.

  - ✓ **Identify Strengths:**
    Recognize your skills and talents that can be further developed or utilized in new ways.

o **Explore New Activities:**
  - ✓ **Hobbies:**
    Try new hobbies or revisit old ones that you enjoy.

  - ✓ **Education:**
    Take courses or attend workshops to learn new skills or expand your knowledge.

o **Personal Development:**
  - ✓ **Mindfulness and meditation:**
    Practice mindfulness or meditation to gain deeper self-awareness.

  - ✓ **Journaling:**
    Keep a journal to explore thoughts and feelings about this life stage.

o **Health and Wellness:**
  - ✓ **Self-care:**
    Prioritize self-care routines, including regular exercises, a balanced diet and adequate sleep.

  - ✓ **Medical Consultation:**
    Regular check-ups with healthcare providers to manage menopausal symptoms effectively.

- o **Reconnect with Passions:**
  - ✓ **Create Pursuits:**
    Engage in creative activities like writing, painting or music.

  - ✓ **Travel:**
    Explore new places and cultures to broaden your horizons and gain fresh perspectives.

- o **Community Involvement:**
  - ✓ **Volunteering:**
    Get involved in community service or volunteer work to give back and find purpose.

  - ✓ **Join Clubs or Groups:**
    Participate in clubs or groups that align with your interests and values.

- o **Set New Life Goals:**
  - ✓ **Short-term Goals:**
    Establish achievable short-term goals to stay motivated.

  - ✓ **Long-term Vision:**
    Create a long-term vision for your future and outline steps to achieve it.

- o **Seek Professional Guidance:**
  - ✓ **Life Coach:**
    Consider working with a life coach to help set goals and navigate this transition.

  - ✓ **Therapist:**
    Seek therapy to address any identity-related issues and develop coping strategies.

o **Embrace Change:**
  - ✓ **Adaptability:**
    Be open to change and willing to adapt to new circumstances and opportunities.

  - ✓ **Positive Mindset:**
    Maintain a positive outlook and focus on the opportunities that come with this new stage of life.

By systematically addressing both empty nest syndrome and need to redefine personal identity, one can navigate menopausal transition with resilience and a renewed sense of purpose.

Therapies for Mental Health Issues:

Menopause can lead to a variety of mental health issues, including depression, anxiety and mood swings. Several therapies are available to address these problems.

Menopause Hormone Therapy (MHT):

MHT, involving estrogen or a combination of estrogen and progesterone, is commonly used to alleviate menopausal symptoms, including hot flashes and mood disturbances. *It can be effective in reducing symptoms of depression and anxiety that are directly related to hormonal changes during menopause.* HRT plays a significant role in addressing various mental health challenges that postmenopausal women may face. The decline in estrogen levels during menopause can lead to various psychological symptoms, including mood swings, anxiety, depression and cognitive disturbances.

Key Roles of MHT in Women's Mental Health:

1. **Mood Stabilization:**
    MHT can help in stabilizing mood swings that are common during the menopausal transition. The therapy may alleviate symptoms of depression and anxiety, improving overall emotional well-being.

2. **Reduction in Depression:**
    Several studies suggest that estrogen therapy, especially when started close to the onset of menopause, can reduce the risk of developing depression in postmenopausal women. Estrogen is thought to influence neurotransmitter systems, such as serotonin, which play a crucial role in mood regulation.

3. **Cognitive Function:**
    There is evidence that MHT may have a protective effect on cognitive function in postmenopausal women. Estrogen is believed to support neural health and may help in preventing the cognitive decline associated with aging and menopause.

4. **Sleep Improvement:**
    Insomnia and other sleep disturbances are common during menopause, often exacerbating mental health issues. MHT can improve sleep quality by reducing hot flashes and night sweats, which in turn can have a positive impact on mental health.

5. **Quality of Life:**
    By addressing the physical and psychological symptoms of menopause, MHT can significantly improve the overall quality of life for postmenopausal women, contributing to better mental health outcomes.

Considerations:

While MHT can be beneficial, it is not suitable for everyone   and may carry certain risks, such as increased risk of breast cancer, blood clots and stroke, depending on individual health profiles. Therefore, the decision to use MHT should be made after thorough investigations for risk involved and consultation with a healthcare provider, considering the potential benefits and the risks based on a woman's health history and preferences.

In conclusion, MHT can be an effective intervention for managing mental health challenges in postmenopausal women, contributing to improved mood, cognitive function and overall wellbeing. However, its use should be personalized and closely monitored.

Non-Hormone Therapies:

o   **Antidepressants**:

Antidepressants particularly selective serotonin reuptake inhibitors **(SSRIs)** and serotonin norepinephrine reuptake inhibitors **(SNRIs)** are often prescribed to manage menopausal symptoms. They can help in mood swings, depression and anxiety. Some of the commonly used antidepressants include:

SSRIs: Fluoxetine, Sertraline and Paroxetine.

SNRIs: Venlafaxine and Desvenlafaxine.

These medications can help stabilize mood and are particularly beneficial for women in whom estrogen is contraindicated or they are not willing to take the same because of side effects.

o   **Antipsychotics:**

Antipsychotics are not generally the first line of treatment for menopause-related mental health issues. They are typically used to manage more severe psychiatric conditions such as bipolar disorder and schizophrenia. However, there may be some specific situations where low doses of certain antipsychotics could be beneficial:

Second-generation antipsychotics (also known as atypical antipsychotics) like quetiapine or olanzapine may be used off-label for severe anxiety or mood disorders, particularly if other treatments have not been effective.

They may help in cases where menopause exacerbates underlying psychiatric conditions (history of severe premenstrual syndrome or postpartum psychosis) and with consultation with psychiatrist.

Effectiveness and Considerations:

The use of antipsychotics for menopause-induced mental health disorders should be approached with caution due to potential side effects, such as weight gain, metabolic syndrome and increased risk of cardiovascular disease. These side effects can be particularly concerning in postmenopausal women.

In summary, while MHT and antidepressants are more commonly used and recommended for managing mental health issues during menopause, antipsychotics might be considered in specific and more severe cases. There use should be carefully monitored by a healthcare provider due to significant side effect profile. It is essential for any treatment plan to be tailored to the individual needs of the patient, taking into account, the severity of symptoms, underlying health conditions and personal preferences.

CHAPTER VII: IMPACT OF BOTH PHYSICAL AND SEXUAL VIOLENCE ON WOMEN'S MENTAL HEALTH

"The moment we begin to fear the opinions of others

and hesitate to tell the truth that is in us, and

from motives of policy are silent when we should speak,

the divine floods of light and life no longer

flow into our souls"

-Elizabeth Cady Stanton (1815 – 1902)

Domestic and work-place violence has long been a major concern for women globally, including in India.

The United Nations defines violence against women as *"any act of gender-based violence that results in physical, sexual or mental harm, including threats of such acts, whether occurring in public or in private life."*

Intimate partner violence:

Intimate partner violence is any behaviour by a spouse that causes physical, sexual or psychological harm. This is one of the most common forms of violence experienced by women globally.

Sexual Violence:

Sexual violence is any sexual act committed against the will of another person, either when this person does not give consent or when consent cannot be given because the person is a child, has mental disability, or is severely intoxicated or unconscious as a result of alcohol or drugs.

Sexual Harassment:

Sexual harassment includes non-contact forms, like sexual comments about person's body parts or appearance, whistling, demands of sexual favors and exposing one's sexual organs at someone. It also includes physical contact forms, like grabbing, pinching, slapping or rubbing against another person in a sexual way.

Human Trafficking:

Human trafficking is the acquisition and exploitation of people, through means, such as force, fraud, coercion, or deception. This heinous crime ensnares millions of women and girls worldwide, many of whom are sexually exploited.

(A) Magnitude of the Problem:

Magnitude of the Problem Globally:

Worldwide, 1 in 3 women have experienced physical or sexual violence – mostly by intimate partner. When accounting for sexual harassment, this figure is even higher.

Worldwide, almost 3 in 5 women were killed by their partners or family in 2017.

> **Source:** Global and regional estimates of violence against women, WHO, 2013;
> Global Study on Homicide 2019, UNODC, 2019.

Worldwide, approximately, 15 million adolescent girls (aged 15 – 19) have experienced forced sex at some point in their life.

Source: *A Familiar Face:*
Violence in the lives of children and adolescents,
UNICEF, 2017.

45% - 55% of women have experienced sexual harassment since the age of 15 in the European Union.

Source: Violence against women:
An EU-wide survey,
European Union Agency for Fundamental Rights,
2014.

72% of all trafficking victims are women and girls. 4 out of 5 trafficked women are trafficked for sexual exploitation.

Source: Global Report on
Trafficking in Persons, UNODC, 2018.

Estimates published by World Health Organization (WHO) indicate that globally about 1 in 3 (30%) of women worldwide have been subjected to either physical and / or sexual intimate partner violence or non-partner sexual violence in their lifetime. Most of this violence is intimate partner violence. (March 2024).

Magnitude of the Problem in India:

Violence against women in India refers to physical or sexual violence include acts such as domestic abuse, sexual assault, acid throwing, forced prostitution, murder (dowry deaths, honor killing).

The safety of working women in India, particularly in urban areas, has been a subject of concern for many years due to the recurrence of heinous crimes. The tragic incident *involving the junior doctor in R. G. Kar Medical College Kolkata recently (August 2024) and the infamous Nirbhaya case (2012)* highlight the gravity of the situation. These reminders are stark reminders of the vulnerabilities that working women face in India.

According to the National Family Health Survey (NFHS), 2019 – 2021, 29.3% of married Indian women between the ages of 18 and 49 years have suffered physical violence; 3.1% of pregnant women aged 18 to 49 have suffered physical violence during their pregnancy (May 24, 2023).

The recurrence of the heinous acts such as sexual and physical assault of junior doctor in Kolkata Medical College, the infamous Nirbhaya case and many others suggest several concerning realities:

Systemic Failures:

These incidents highlight the persistent failures in our legal and judicial systems; where delayed justice, inadequate protection for victims and lack of stringent punishments for perpetrators contribute to the recurrence of such crimes.

Cultural and Societal Attitudes:

The recurrence of these acts underscores deeply ingrained cultural and societal attitudes towards women, where patriarchal norms and gender inequality continue to prevail.

This toxic mindset perpetuates a cycle of violence and impurity.

Gaps in Law Enforcement:

The inability of law enforcement agencies to effectively prevent such crimes and protect potential victims points to significant gaps in policing, surveillance and community safety measures.

Lack of Public Awareness and Education:

These incidences also suggest a failure in public education and awareness campaigns aimed at changing societal attitudes towards women, promoting gender equality and preventing violence.

Need for Systemic Change:

The recurrence of such heinous acts indicates an urgent need for systemic change, including comprehensive reforms in law enforcement, judicial processes, public education and societal norms to ensure the safety and dignity of all individuals, particularly women.

(B)Factors Responsible for Such Incidents:

1. Patriarchal Mindset:

Deeply ingrained patriarchal attitudes often perpetuate the notion that women are subordinate to men, which can lead to misogynistic behavior, including violence. This mindset can influence how women are treated both in public and private places.

2. Lack of Effective Law Enforcement:

Although laws exist to protect women, the implementation and enforcement of these laws can be inadequate. Delays in justice, lenient sentences and corruption within the law enforcement agencies contribute a culture of impurity.

Delayed justice can exacerbate the trauma and suffering of the victim. The uncertainty and prolonged wait for a decision can have severe psychological and emotional impacts. *I appreciate the role of the Supreme Court, and High Courts in taking Suo motu cognizance of some such brutal rape cases, addressing the issues, and leading to law, and policy changes.* The criminalization of politics and politicization of the police system lead to delay in filing first information reports (FIR), and influence the crime investigation, allowing criminals to go unpunished, raising concerns of a public safety threat by criminals remaining free.

3. Cultural Norms and Victim Blaming:

Societal norms that blame victims rather than perpetrators can discourage women from reporting crimes. Fear of stigmatization or retaliation can lead underreporting allowing perpetuators to go unpunished.

4. Inadequate Public Sector Infrastructure:

Lack of security in working places, inadequate public transportation security and insufficient police presence in vulnerable areas make it easier for such crimes to occur.

5.Media Representation:

Media often sensationalizes violence against women without adequately addressing the root causes. This can desensitize the public and sometimes even glorify the criminals.

6.Gender Inequality and Economic Dependency:

Economic dependence on male counterparts can make women more vulnerable to exploitation and violence. Gender inequalities in work places, where women may not feel empowered to speak up against harassment, again contribute to the problem.

7.Educational and Awareness Gaps:

Lack of comprehensive education on gender equality and respect for women's rights from an early age contributes to the persistence of sexist attitudes and behaviors.

8.Social and Economic Disparities:

Disparities in social and economic status can exacerbate the vulnerability of women to violence, as those from marginalized communities may have fewer resources to seek justice.

(C) Addressing the Issue:

1.Strengthening Law Enforcement:

Ensuring swift and stringent action against perpetrators, improving the training and sensitivity of law enforcement personnel, and making the legal process more accessible to victims are crucial steps.

The criminalization of politics and politicization of the police system should be reduced to minimum so that there will not be delay in filing first information reports (FIR).

2.Public Awareness and Education:

Raising awareness about gender equality and respect for women through education and media campaigns can help change societal attitudes over time.

3.Empowerng Women Economically:

Enhancing opportunity for women in education and employment, ensuring equal pay, and supporting women entrepreneurs can reduce economic dependence and vulnerability.

4.Improving Public Infrastructure:

Investing in safer public places, better lighting, reliable public transportation, and increasing the presence of security personnel can deter crimes.

5.Support System for Victims:

Establishing robust support systems for victims, including legal aid, counseling and safe houses, can encourage more women to come forward and seek justice.

The safety of working women in India remains a complex issue that requires a multifaceted approach, involving legal, political, societal and cultural changes. Only through concerted efforts at all levels of society, can meaningful process be made in ensuring that woman can work and live without fear.

(D) Impact of Such Incidents on Women's Life:

Incidences of sexual violence and brutal crimes against women, like the one that happened recently with the junior doctor of R.G. Medical College Kolkata, in the past the Nirbhaya case and many more such cases occurring recurrently; have profound and far-reaching impact on mental health of women, both directly and indirectly. The psychological toll can be devastating and enduring, affecting not only the victims but also the broader female population who live in fear of such of violence.

"Violence has immediate effects on women's Health, which in cases is fatal. Physical, mental and behavioral health consequences can also persist long after the violence has stopped."

-World Health Organization (WHO)

Direct Impact on Victims:

1.Post-traumatic stress disorder (PTSD)

Victims of sexual violence often develop PTSD, characterized by flashbacks, nightmares, severe anxiety and uncomfortable thoughts about the incident. This can severely impair their ability to function in daily life.

2.Depression:

Feelings of hopelessness, sadness and a loss of interest in life are common among survivors. Depression can lead to difficulties in maintaining relationships, job performance and overall quality of life.

3.Anxiety Disorders:

Survivors may experience heightened level of anxiety, leading to panic attacks, social withdrawal and an overwhelming sense of fear. This can make it difficult for them to trust others or feel safe in their environment.

4.Self-Blame and Guilt:

Victims often internalize societal victim-blaming attitudes, which can lead to feelings of guilt and self-blame. This exacerbates mental health issues, as they may feel responsible for the violence inflicted upon them.

5.Substace Abuse:

To cope with psychological pain, some victims may turn to alcohol or drugs, which can lead to substance abuse problems and further deteriorate their mental and physical health.

6.Suicidal Thoughts and Behavior:

The overwhelming psychological distress caused by such incidents can lead some survivors to contemplate or attempt suicide.

Indirect Impact on the Broader Female Population:

1.Hightened Sense of Fear and Insecurity:

Women in general may develop a pervasive sense of fear and insecurity, especially when they are alone or in unfamiliar environments. This can lead to hypervigilance and increased anxiety, affecting their ability to live freely and confidently.

2.Restricted Mobility and Lifestyle Changes:

Fear of similar attacks can cause women to limit their movements, avoid certain places, or change their routines, which can lead to social isolation and reduced opportunities for personal and professional growth.

3. Impact on Professional Life:

The fear of violence can make it difficult for women to peruse certain carriers, work late hours or travel for work, which can limit their professional opportunities and lead to economic disadvantages.

4.Impact on Mental Health of Loved Ones:

The mental health of victim's family and friends can also be severely impacted, leading to widespread emotional distress within the community.

5.Social Trauma:

Repeated incidents of sexual violence contribute to a collective trauma among women in society, where the constant threat of violence becomes a heavy psychological burden. This can also lead to a breakdown in trust within the community and between genders.

6.Normalization of Fear:

Over time, fear of sexual violence can become so normalized that it's seen as an expected part of being a woman in society. This normalization can have a chilling effect on women's mental health, making anxiety and fear constant companions.

Long-Term Consequences:

1.Intergenerational Impact:

The trauma from such incidents can be passed down to future generations as mothers who have experienced violence or live in fear may unintentionally transfer their anxiety and fear to their children.

2.Impact on Society's Mental Health:

A society where women are constantly in fear cannot thrive. The overall mental health of the community suffers, leading to a culture where anxiety, mistrust and fear are pervasive.

The impact on such incidents on the mental health of women is profound, creating a ripple effect that extends far beyond the immediate victim. Addressing these mental health consequences requires not only supporting survivors through comprehensive mental health services but also creating a societal shift that prioritizes a safety, dignity and well-being of women.

(E) Domestic Violence:

Domestic violence in relation to dowry, remains a significant issue that affects women's mental health deeply. When a woman is subjected to abuse by her husband or family members, particularly in relation to dowry demands, it often leads to severe psychological trauma. This type of violence can manifest in physical, emotional and economic abuse, creating an environment of constant fear, anxiety and helplessness.

The impact on mental health can be profound and long-lasting. Women in such situations often express depression, anxiety disorders, post-traumatic stress disorder (PTSD), and in severe cases, suicidal tendencies. The stress of dealing with ongoing abuse can also lead to psychosomatic disorders, where the body begins to exhibit physical symptoms due to mental strain. For instance, chronic headaches, gastrointestinal issues and common disturbances are common among victims.

Moreover, the stigma associated with domestic violence, especially when it involves dowry, often prevents women from seeking help. The fear of societal judgement, the potential loss of family honor and economic dependency make it difficult for women to escape these situations. This isolation exacerbates the mental health issues, as women feel trapped and unsupported.

Intervention strategies must involve both legal and psychological support. Legal avenues should be made accessible to women to help them fight against such violence, while psychological counseling is crucial to help them recover from the trauma. Creating awareness and breaking the silence around dowry-related domestic violence is essential to protect women's mental health and ensure their well-being.

CHAPTER VIII: CONCLUSION

"No one saves us but ourselves.

No one can and no one may.

We ourselves must walk the path"

-Buddha

According to the **American Psychiatric Association,** each year, one in five women in the United States has a mental health problem such as depression, post-traumatic stress disorder (PTSD). There are many other challenges women can face with their mental health and emotional wellness.

Studies show that, **"Women are more than twice as likely as men to get an anxiety disorder in their lifetime."** In addition, women may face challenges with their hormones, reproductive mental health, and being victims of abuse.

Domestic and work-place violence has long been a major concern for women globally, including in India.

So if you feel like you are struggling right now, you're not alone. And sometimes, we can all benefit from some encouragement, inspiration and even a gentle nudge in a helpful direction.

Thankfully, we can learn from the experiences and stories of others. Their tips and encouragement can help keep you motivated, probe wisdom to help you navigate your situation and positively shift your thinking.

Unraveling Women's Mental Health across Life Stages:

Adolescence:

- **Challenges:**
  Adolescence brings hormonal changes, identify formation, peer pressure and academic stress. These factors can lead to issues such as depression, anxiety, eating disorders and body image concerns.

- **Interventions:**
  Early mental health education, supportive family and social environments, access to counseling services, and fostering healthy lifestyle habits.

- **Strategies for Mental Health:**
  o Encourage open communication about feelings and mental health.

  o Promote self-esteem and positive body image through education and support.

  o Implement school-based mental health programs.

Reproductive Age Group:

- **Challenges:**
  This stage encompasses significant life events like pregnancy, childbirth, and the balancing of career and family issues include perinatal depression, anxiety, postpartum depression and the stress of multiple roles.

- **Interventions:**
  Comprehensive prenatal and postnatal care, mental health screening, support groups and flexible work policies.

- **Strategies for Mental Health:**

  - o Regular screening for mental issues during and after pregnancy.

  - o Education and support for new mothers on recognizing and seeking help for postpartum depression.

  - o Supportive policies at work to balance career and family responsibilities.

Midlife/Menopausal Age Group:

- **Challenges:**
  Midlife brings menopause, career transitions and possibly caring for aging parents or experiencing the empty nest syndrome. Symptoms may include mood swings, depression and cognitive changes.

- **Interventions:**
  Hormone replacement therapy (if appropriate), cognitive-behavioral therapy, mindfulness practices and community support.

- **Strategies for Mental Health:**
  - o Educate women about menopausal symptoms and available treatments.

  - o Promote regular physical activity and healthy eating to manage symptoms.

  - o Provide access to mental health services and support networks.

General Strategies to Maintain Mental Health across All Stages:

- **Education and Awareness:**
  Increase awareness about mental health issues specific to each life stage and educate women on how to recognize symptoms and seek help.

- **Support Systems:**
  Foster strong social support networks, including family, friends and community resources.

- **Access to Care:**
  Ensure access to mental health services, including counseling, therapy and psychiatric care, tailored to women's unique needs at each stage of life.

- **Healthy Lifestyles:**
  Encourage a healthy lifestyle through regular exercise, balanced nutrition, adequate sleep and stress management techniques.

- **Work-Life Balance:**
  Promote policies and practices that support work-life balance, flexible working hours and parental leave.

- **Mental Health Policies:**
  Advocate for mental health policies that address the unique needs of women and provide funding for research and support services.

By understanding and addressing the specific mental health challenges women face at different stages of their lives, we can promote a holistic approach to well-being, ensuring that women receive the support and care they need to thrive.

Lastly, to combat Sexual and Physical Violence Against Women:

It requires a multifaceted approach. Here are the key actions:

1. **Legal Reforms and Enforcement:**
   Strengthen law against sexual and physical violence and timely justice for victims.

2. **Education and Awareness:**
   Implement comprehensive educational programs that challenge harmful gender norms and promote respect for women's right from an early age.

3. **Support Systems:**
   Establish and expand support services for victims, including hot lines, shelters, legal aid and psychological counseling.

4. **Community Involvement:**
   Encourage community-based interventions and support networks that actively work to prevent violence and to protect women.

5. **Empowerment and Economic Independence:**
   Promote women's economic empowerment through education, job opportunities and support for women entrepreneurs, reducing their dependency.

These actions when combined, can create a safer environment for women and significantly reduce the incidence of violence.

CHAPTER IX: REFERENCES:

1.Is psychopathology associated with the timing of pubertal development?
Journal of the American Academy of Child & Adolescent Psychiatry. (1997) J.A. Graber *et al.*

2.Is pubertal timing associated with psychopathology in young adulthood
Journal of the American Academy of Child & Adolescent Psychiatry (2004) A.F. Jorm *et al.*

3.Association of obesity with anxiety, depression and emotional well-being: a community survey
Australian & New Zealand Journal of Public Health
(2003)   R. Kaltiala-Heino *et al.*

4.Early puberty is associated with mental health problems in middle adolescence
Social Science & Medicine
(2003)L. Lien *et al.*

5.The relationship between age of menarche and mental distress in Norwegian adolescent girls and girls from different immigrant groups in Norway: results from an urban city cross-sectional survey
Social Science & Medicine (2006) R.S. Lipman *et al.*

6.The Hopkins symptom checklist (HSCL)–factors derived from the HSCL-90
Journal of Affective Disorders (1979) J.M. Siegel *et al.*

7.Body image, perceived pubertal timing, and adolescent mental health
Journal of Adolescent Health (1999) A.J. Zametkin *et al.*

8.Psychiatric aspects of child and adolescent obesity: a review of the past 10 years

Journal of the American Academy of Child & Adolescent Psychiatry (2004)

9.Holm-Denoma, J. M., Hankin, B. L., & Young, J. F. (2014). Developmental trends of eating disorder symptoms and comorbid internalizing symptoms in children and adolescents. *Eating Behaviors, 15*(2), 275–279. https://doi.org/10.1016/j.eatbeh.2014.03.015

Article PubMed Central Google Scholar

10.Impett, E. A., Henson, J. M., Breines, J. G., Schooler, D., & Tolman, D. L. (2011). Embodiment feels better: Girls' body objectification and well-being across adolescence. *Psychology of Women Quarterly, 35*(1), 46–58. https://doi.org/10.1177/0361684310391641

Article Google Scholar

11.Ivie, E. J., Pettitt, A., Moses, L. J., & Allen, N. B. (2020). A meta-analysis of the association between adolescent social media use and depressive symptoms. *Journal of Affective Disorders, 275,* 165–174. https://doi.org/10.1016/j.jad.2020.06.014

Article PubMed Google Scholar

12.Jarman, H. K., Marques, M. D., McLean, S. A., Slater, A., & Paxton, S. J. (2021). Social media, body satisfaction and well-being among adolescents: A mediation model of appearance-ideal internalization and comparison. *Body Image, 36,* 139–148. https://doi.org/10.1016/j.bodyim.2020.11.005

Article PubMed Google Scholar

13.Johnson, B. K., Potocki, B., & Veldhuis, J. (2019). Is that my friend or an advert? The effectiveness of Instagram native advertisements posing as social posts. *Journal of Computer-Mediated Communication, 24*(3), 108–125. https://doi.org/10.1093/jcmc/zmz003

Article **Google Scholar**

14.Jones, D. C. (2001). Social comparison and body image: Attractiveness comparisons to models and peers among adolescent girls and boys. *Sex Roles, 45*(9), 645–664. https://doi.org/10.1023/A:1014815725852

Article **Google Scholar**

15.Jones, D. C., Vigfusdottir, T. H., & Lee, Y. (2004). Body image and the appearance culture among adolescent girls and boys: An examination of friend conversations, peer criticism, appearance magazines, and the internalization of appearance ideals. *Journal of Adolescent Research, 19*(3), 323–339. https://doi.org/10.1177/0743558403258847

Article **Google Scholar**

17.Jones, L. R., Fries, E., & Danish, S. J. (2007). Gender and ethnic differences in body image and opposite sex figure preferences of rural adolescents. *Body Image, 4*(1), 103–108. https://doi.org/10.1016/j.bodyim.2006.11.005

Article **PubMed** **PubMed Central** **Google Scholar**

18.Kapidzic, S., & Herring, S. C. (2015). Race, gender, and self-presentation in teen profile photographs. *New Media & Society, 17*(6), 958–976. https://doi.org/10.1177/1461444813520301

Article **Google Scholar**

19.Keyes, K. M., Gary, D., O'Malley, P. M., Hamilton, A., & Schulenberg, J. (2019). Recent increases in depressive symptoms among U.S. adolescents: Trends from 1991 to 2018. *Social Psychiatry and Psychiatric Epidemiology, 54*(8), 987–996. https://doi.org/10.1007/s00127-019-01697-8

Article **PubMed** **PubMed Central** **Google Scholar**

20.Kim, H. M. (2020). What do others' reactions to body posting on Instagram tell us? The effects of social media comments on viewers' body image perception. *New Media & Society*. https://doi.org/10.1177/1461444820956368 **ArticleGoogle Scholar**

21.Pfeifer, J.H.; Allen, N.B. Puberty Initiates Cascading Relationships Between Neurodevelopmental, Social, and Internalizing Processes Across Adolescence. *Biol. Psychiatry* **2021**, *89*, 99–108. [**Google Scholar**] [**CrossRef**]

22.Guo, N.; Robakis, T.; Miller, C.; Butwick, A. Prevalence of Depression Among Women of Reproductive Age in the United States. *Obstet. Gynecol.* **2018**, *131*, 671–679. [**Google Scholar**] [**CrossRef**]

23.Angold, A.; Costello, E.J.; Erkanli, A.; Worthman, C.M. Pubertal Changes in Hormone Levels and Depression in Girls. *Psychol. Med.* **1999**, *29*, 1043–1053. [**Google Scholar**] [**CrossRef**] [**PubMed**]

24.Gordon, J.L.; Eisenlohr-Moul, T.A.; Rubinow, D.R.; Schrubbe, L.; Girdler, S.S. Naturally Occurring Changes in Estradiol Concentrations in the Menopause Transition Predict Morning Cortisol and Negative Mood in Perimenopausal Depression. *Clin. Psychol. Sci.* **2016**, *4*, 919–935. [**Google Scholar**] [**CrossRef**] [**PubMed**]

25.Bennett, H.A.; Einarson, A.; Taddio, A.; Koren, G.; Einarson, T.R. Prevalence of Depression during Pregnancy: Systematic Review. *Obstet. Gynecol.* **2004**, *103*, 698–709. [**Google Scholar**] [**CrossRef**] [**PubMed**]

26.Bloch, M.; Schmidt, P.J.; Danaceau, M.; Murphy, J.; Nieman, L.; Rubinow, D.R. Effects of Gonadal Steroids in Women with a History of Postpartum Depression. *Am. J. Psychiatry* **2000**, *157*, 924–930. [**Google Scholar**] [**CrossRef**]

27.Georgakis, M.K.; Thomopoulos, T.P.; Diamantaras, A.-A.; Kalogirou, E.I.; Skalkidou, A.; Daskalopoulou, S.S.; Petridou,

E.T. Association of Age at Menopause and Duration of Reproductive Period With Depression After Menopause: A Systematic Review and Meta-Analysis. *JAMA Psychiatry* **2016**, *73*, 139–149. [**Google Scholar**] [**CrossRef**]

28.Freeman, E.W.; Sammel, M.D.; Liu, L.; Gracia, C.R.; Nelson, D.B.; Hollander, L. Hormones and Menopausal Status as Predictors of Depression in Women in Transition to Menopause. *Arch. Gen. Psychiatry* **2004**, *61*, 62–70. [**Google Scholar**] [**CrossRef**]
Gordon, J.L.; Peltier, A.; Grummisch, J.A.; Sykes Tottenham, L. Estradiol Fluctuation, Sensitivity to Stress, and Depressive Symptoms in the Menopause Transition: A Pilot Study. *Front. Psychol.* **2019**, *10*, 1319. [**Google Scholar**] [**CrossRef**]

29.Gordon, J.L.; Rubinow, D.R.; Eisenlohr-Moul, T.A.; Leserman, J.; Girdler, S.S. Estradiol Variability, Stressful Life Events, and the Emergence of Depressive Symptomatology during the Menopausal Transition. *Menopause* **2016**, *23*, 257–266. [**Google Scholar**] [**CrossRef**]

30.Almeida, O.P.; Lautenschlager, N.; Vasikaram, S.; Leedman, P.; Flicker, L. Association between Physiological Serum Concentration of Estrogen and the Mental Health of Community-Dwelling Postmenopausal Women Age 70 Years and over. *Am. J. Geriatr. Psychiatry* **2005**, *13*, 142–149. [**Google Scholar**] [**CrossRef**]

31.Ryan, J.; Burger, H.G.; Szoeke, C.; Lehert, P.; Ancelin, M.-L.; Henderson, V.W.; Dennerstein, L. A Prospective Study of the Association between Endogenous Hormones and Depressive Symptoms in Postmenopausal Women. *Menopause* **2009**, *16*, 509–517. [**Google Scholar**] [**CrossRef**]

32.Gudipally, P.R.; Sharma, G.K. *Premenstrual Syndrome*; StatPearls Publishing: Treasure Island, FL, USA, 2022. [**Google Scholar**]

33.Roomruangwong, C.; Carvalho, A.F.; Comhaire, F.; Maes, M. Lowered Plasma Steady-State Levels of Progesterone Combined With Declining Progesterone Levels During the Luteal Phase Predict Peri-Menstrual Syndrome and Its Major Subdomains. *Front. Psychol.* **2019**, *10*, 2446. [Google Scholar] [CrossRef] [PubMed]

34.Ford, O.; Lethaby, A.; Roberts, H.; Mol, B.W.J. Progesterone for Premenstrual Syndrome. *Cochrane Database Syst. Rev.* **2012**, *2012*, CD003415. [Google Scholar] [CrossRef] [PubMed]

35.Lovick, T.A.; Guapo, V.G.; Anselmo-Franci, J.A.; Loureiro, C.M.; Faleiros, M.C.M.; Del Ben, C.M.; Brandão, M.L. A Specific Profile of Luteal Phase Progesterone Is Associated with the Development of Premenstrual Symptoms. *Psychoneuroendocrinology* **2017**, *75*, 83–90. [Google Scholar] [CrossRef] [PubMed]
Epperson, C.N.; Pittman, B.; Czarkowski, K.A.; Stiklus, S.; Krystal, J.H.; Grillon, C. Luteal-Phase Accentuation of Acoustic Startle Response in Women with Premenstrual Dysphoric Disorder. *Neuropsychopharmacology* **2007**, *32*, 2190–2198. [Google Scholar] [CrossRef]

36.Hantsoo, L.; Epperson, C.N. Premenstrual Dysphoric Disorder: Epidemiology and Treatment. *Curr. Psychiatry Rep.* **2015**, *17*, 87. [Google Scholar] [CrossRef] [PubMed]

37.Ko, C.-H.; Long, C.-Y.; Yen, C.-F.; Chen, C.-S.; Wang, P.-W.; Yen, J.-Y. Gonadotrophic Hormone and Reinforcement Sensitivity Systems in Women with Premenstrual Dysphoric Disorder. *Psychiatry Clin. Neurosci.* **2014**, *68*, 785–794. [Google Scholar] [CrossRef]

38.Yen, J.-Y.; Lin, H.-C.; Lin, P.-C.; Liu, T.-L.; Long, C.-Y.; Ko, C.-H. Early- and Late-Luteal-Phase Estrogen and Progesterone Levels of Women with Premenstrual Dysphoric Disorder. *Int. J. Environ. Res. Public Health* **2019**, *16*, 4352. [Google Scholar] [CrossRef]

39.Sacher, J.; Zsido, R.G.; Barth, C.; Zientek, F.; Rullmann, M.; Luthardt, J.; Patt, M.; Becker, G.A.; Rusjan, P.; Witte, A.V.; et al. Increase in Serotonin Transporter Binding in Patients With Premenstrual Dysphoric Disorder Across the Menstrual Cycle: A Case-Control Longitudinal Neuroreceptor Ligand Positron Emission Tomography Imaging Study. *Biol. Psychiatry* **2023**, *93*, 1081–1088. [**Google Scholar**] [**CrossRef**]

40.Nillni, Y.I.; Rasmusson, A.M.; Paul, E.L.; Pineles, S.L. The Impact of the Menstrual Cycle and Underlying Hormones in Anxiety and PTSD: What Do We Know and Where Do We Go From Here? *Curr. Psychiatry Rep.* **2021**, *23*, 8. [**Google Scholar**] [**CrossRef**]

41.McLeod, D.R.; Hoehn-Saric, R.; Foster, G.V.; Hipsley, P.A. The Influence of Premenstrual Syndrome on Ratings of Anxiety in Women with Generalized Anxiety Disorder. *Acta Psychiatr. Scand.* **1993**, *88*, 248–251. [**Google Scholar**] [**CrossRef**]

42.Veen, J.F.V.; Jonker, B.W.; Vliet, I.M.V.; Zitman, F.G. The effects of female reproductive hormones in generalized social anxiety disorder. *Int J Psychiatry Med.* **2009**, *39*, 283–295.

43. Girls Not Brides. Child Marriage Around the World [Internet]. Child Marriage Around the World; 2017. Available from: https://www.girlsnotbrides.org/where-does-it-happen/

44.. UNICEF. Child marriage: Latest trends and future prospects. New York; 2017.

45. Rasmussen B, Maharaj N, Karan A, Symons J, Selvaraj S, Kumar R, et al. Evaluating interventions to reduce child marriage in India. *J Glob Heal Reports*. 2021;5. [Google Scholar]

46. Zaman M, Koski A. Child marriage in Canada: A systematic review. *PLoS One*. 2020;15(3):3. doi:

10.1371/journal.pone.0229676 [PMC free article] [PubMed] [CrossRef] [Google Scholar]

47.. Kalamar AM, Lee-Rife S, Hindin MJ. Interventions to Prevent Child Marriage Among Young People in Low- and Middle-Income Countries: A Systematic Review of the Published and Gray Literature. *J Adolesc Heal.* 2016;59(3):S16–21. doi: 10.1016/j.jadohealth.2016.06.015 [PubMed] [CrossRef] [Google Scholar]

48. Henderson R. Ending child marriage by 2030: Tracking progress and identifying gap. [online] World Vision UK [Internet]. Girls Not Brides. 2016. Available from: https://www.girlsnotbrides.org/documents/464/Ending_Child_Marriage_by_2030.pdf

49. Wodon Q, Nguyen MC, Tsimpo C. Child Marriage, Education, and Agency in Uganda. *Fem Econ.* 2016;22(1):54–79. [Google Scholar]

50. Ashraf S, Abrar-ul-haq M, Ashraf S. Domestic Violence against Women: Empirical Evidence from Pakistan. *Pertanika J Soc Sci.* 2017;25:3. [Google Scholar]

51 Godha D, Hotchkiss DR, Gage AJ. Association between child marriage and reproductive health outcomes and service utilization: A multi-country study from south Asia. *J Adolesc Heal.* 2013;52(5):552–8. doi: 10.1016/j.jadohealth.2013.01.021 [PubMed] [CrossRef] [Google Scholar]

52. Raj A, Boehmer U. Girl child marriage and its association with national rates of HIV, maternal health, and infant mortality across 97 countries. *Violence Against Women.* 2013;19(4):536–51. doi: 10.1177/1077801213487747 [PubMed] [CrossRef] [Google Scholar]

Rodabaugh B, Austin M. New York: Garland Press; 1981. Sexual assault. [Google Scholar]

53. Kumari R. Rural female adolescence: Indian scenario. *Soc Change.* 1995;25:177–88. [PubMed] [Google Scholar]

54. Levine S, Koenig J. London: WH Allen; 1983. Why men rape: Interviews with convicted rapists. [Google Scholar]

55. Herbert TW. Cambridge: Harvard University Press; 2002. Sexual violence and American manhood. Illustrated ed. [Google Scholar]

56. Zimmerling R. International University Bremen: AK Interkultureller Demokratievergleich; 2003. Jun, 'Guilt Cultures' vs 'Shame Cultures': Political Implications? Paper given at the International Conference on Reassessing Democracy: New Approaches to Governance, Citizenship and Multiple Identities in Comparative Research; pp. 20–21. [Google Scholar]

57. Hofstede G. Thousand Oaks, CA: Sage; 2001. Culture's consequences: Comparing values, behaviors, institutions, and organizations across nations. [Google Scholar]

58. Campbell R, Ahrens CE, Sefl T, Wasco SM, Barnes HE. Social reactions to rape victims: Healing and hurtful effects on psychological and physical health outcomes. *Violence Vict.* 2001;16:287–302. [PubMed] [Google Scholar]

59. Lonsway KA, Fitzgerald LF. Rape myths: In review. *Psychol Women Q.* 1994;18:133–64. [Google Scholar]

60. Pedersen SH, Strömwall LA. Victim Blame, Sexism and Just-World Beliefs: A Cross-Cultural Comparison. *Psychiatry Psychol Law.* 2013. [Last accessed date on 2013 June 5]. Available from: http://dx.doi.org/10.1080/13218719.2013.770715 .

61.Sapkota D, Baird K, Saito A, Anderson D. Interventions for reducing and/or controlling domestic violence among pregnant women in low- and middle-income countries: a systematic review. Syst Rev. 2019 Apr 02;8(1):79. [PMC free article] [PubMed]

62.Klein LB, Chesworth BR, Howland-Myers JR, Rizo CF, Macy RJ. Housing Interventions for Intimate Partner

Violence Survivors: A Systematic Review. Trauma Violence Abuse. 2021 Apr;22(2):249-264. [PubMed]

63. Marie-Mitchell A, Kostolansky R. A Systematic Review of Trials to Improve Child Outcomes Associated With Adverse Childhood Experiences. Am J Prev Med. 2019 May;56(5):756-764. [PubMed]

64. Lewis NV, Dowrick A, Sohal A, Feder G, Griffiths C. Implementation of the Identification and Referral to Improve Safety programme for patients with experience of domestic violence and abuse: A theory-based mixed-method process evaluation. Health Soc Care Community. 2019 Jul;27(4):e298-e312. [PMC free article] [PubMed]

65. Sarkar R, Ozanne-Smith J, Bassed R. Systematic Review of the Patterns of Orofacial Injuries in Physically Abused Children and Adolescents. Trauma Violence Abuse. 2021 Jan;22(1):136-146. [PubMed]

66. Gao S, Assink M, Liu T, Chan KL, Ip P. Associations Between Rejection Sensitivity, Aggression, and Victimization: A Meta-Analytic Review. Trauma Violence Abuse. 2021 Jan;22(1):125-135. [PubMed]
        7.
67. Zeppegno P, Gramaglia C, di Marco S, Guerriero C, Consol C, Loreti L, Martelli M, Marangon D, Carli V, Sarchiapone M. Intimate Partner Homicide Suicide: a Mini-Review of the Literature (2012-2018). Curr Psychiatry Rep. 2019 Feb 21;21(3):13. [PubMed]
        8.
68. Hackenberg EAM, Sallinen V, Handolin L, Koljonen V. Victims of Severe Intimate Partner Violence Are Left Without Advocacy Intervention in Primary Care Emergency Rooms: A Prospective Observational Study. J Interpers Violence. 2021 Aug;36(15-16):7832-7854. [PubMed]

69.Gottlieb A, Mahabir M. The Effect of Multiple Types of Intimate Partner Violence on Maternal Criminal Justice Involvement. J Interpers Violence. 2021 Jul;36(13-14):6797-6820. [PubMed]

70.Roscoe LA, Schenck DP. Victim of Abuse, or Bully? The Case of the 800-Pound Man. Narrat Inq Bioeth. 2018;8(3):261-271. [PubMed]

71.Wahi A, Zaleski KL, Lampe J, Bevan P, Koski A. The Lived Experience of Child Marriage in the United States. Soc Work Public Health. 2019;34(3):201-213. [PubMed]

72.Harland KK, Peek-Asa C, Saftlas AF. Intimate Partner Violence and Controlling Behaviors Experienced by Emergency Department Patients: Differences by Sexual Orientation and Gender Identification. J Interpers Violence. 2021 Jun;36(11-12):NP6125-NP6143. [PMC free article] [PubMed]

73.Jiang Y, DeBare D, Colomer I, Wesley J, Seaberry J, Viner-Brown S. Characteristics of Victims and Suspects in Domestic Violence-Related Homicide - Rhode Island Violent Death Reporting System, 2004-2015. R I Med J (2013). 2018 Dec 03;101(10):58-61. [PubMed]

74.Stone LB, Amole MC, Cyranowski JM, Swartz HA. History of childhood emotional abuse predicts lower resting-state high-frequency heart rate variability in depressed women. Psychiatry Res. 2018 Nov;269:681-687. [PMC free article] [PubMed]

75.Hansen JB, Killough EF, Moffatt ME, Knapp JF. Retinal Hemorrhages: Abusive Head Trauma or Not? Pediatr Emerg Care. 2018 Sep;34(9):665-670. [PubMed]

76.Skott S. Disaggregating Violence: Understanding the Decline. J Interpers Violence. 2021 Aug;36(15-16):7670-7694. [PubMed]

77.Lifflander AL. Hard Times and Hard Stops. JAMA. 2019 Mar 05;321(9):837-838. [PubMed]

78.Saywitz KJ, Wells CR, Larson RP, Hobbs SD. Effects of Interviewer Support on Children's Memory and Suggestibility: Systematic Review and Meta-Analyses of Experimental Research. Trauma Violence Abuse. 2019 Jan;20(1):22-39. [PubMed]

79.Jordan KS, Steelman SH, Leary M, Varela-Gonzalez L, Lassiter SL, Montminy L, Bellow EF. Pediatric Sexual Abuse: An Interprofessional Approach to Optimizing Emergency Care. J Forensic Nurs. 2019 Jan/Mar;15(1):18-25. [PubMed]

80.US Preventive Services Task Force. Curry SJ, Krist AH, Owens DK, Barry MJ, Caughey AB, Davidson KW, Doubeni CA, Epling JW, Grossman DC, Kemper AR, Kubik M, Landefeld CS, Mangione CM, Silverstein M, Simon MA, Tseng CW, Wong JB.

Previous Books Published in the series "Women's Health"

All books are available on Amazon.in as well as on Amazon.com. Universal link is given below:

Universal Link for All Books:

https://relinks.me/B0BW6ZVMXY

1. Preconception Care Makes A Difference

"Preconception Care and Counselling is the window of opportunity to tackle all unhealthy maternal problems resulting in favorable environment for the growth of embryo/fetus."

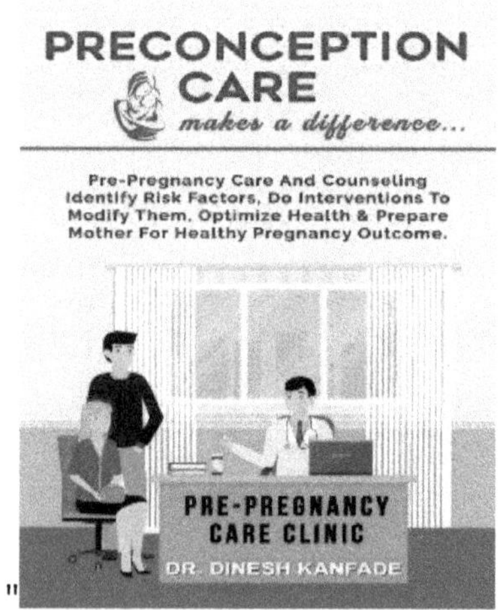

2.   Understanding Menopause

"The biggest achievement of the last century is greater longevity that has resulted in an increased aged population worldwide. But the advantage of increased longevity is only when it is translated into healthy aging. Discover the secrets for understanding and managing menopause, thereby improving quality of life with this comprehensive updated guide."

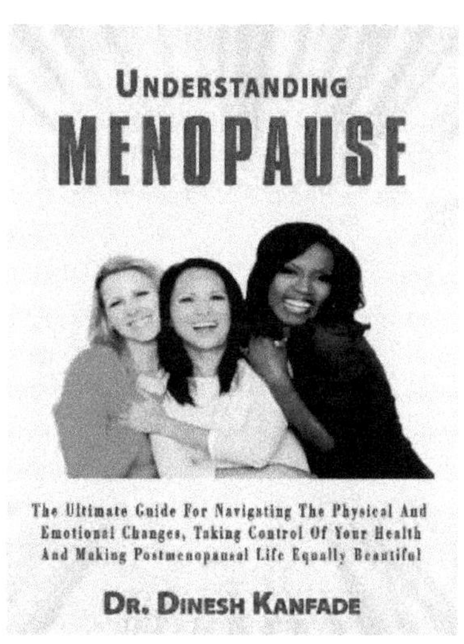

3. Heart and Bone Health

"We are living in aged population worldwide. It is obvious that women live significant part of their life after menopause. The ovaries of long years of dedicated service, have not the ability of retiring gracefully. But because of estrogen deficiency, ovaries become irritable and transmits this irritation to various organs of the body resulting in non-communicable diseases such as cardiovascular disease and osteoporosis. The advantage of increased longevity is only when it is translated into healthy aging. With a healthy lifestyle and understanding the pathophysiology of cardiovascular disease and osteoporosis in postmenopausal women, not only years will be added to increase the lifespan, but the extra years added will be of good quality. Discover the secretes of managing heart and bone health in postmenopausal women, thereby improving quality of life with this comprehensive guide."

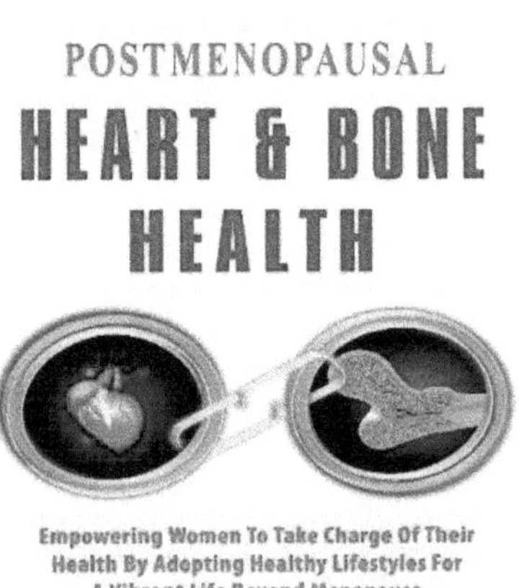

4. Embracing Postmenopausal Intimacy

"The postmenopausal phase, with its unique challenges and opportunities stands as a testament to the resilience of human intimacy. It is within this period of transformation that find an invitation to redefine and to rediscover physical closeness. Don't miss out on the transformative wisdom within these pages. Embrace the journey towards vibrant and fulfilling postmenopausal intimacy."

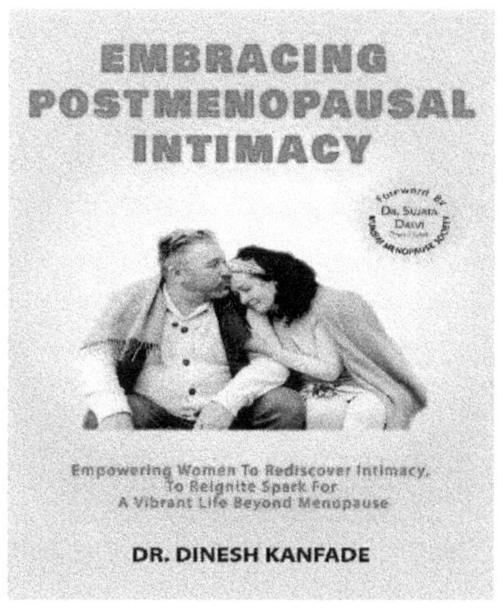

5. Menstrual Health and Hygiene

The stigma surrounding menstruation has a significant impact on women and girls worldwide. It can lead to feelings of shame, embarrassment, lack of confidence and social isolation, which can result in poor menstrual hygiene practices and a lack of access to menstrual products. Poor menstrual hygiene can have disastrous consequences, including health risks such as cervical cancer, reproductive tract infections, urinary tract infections and toxic shock syndrome. Additionally, the stigma can affect educational opportunities for girls, causing missed school days due to a lack of adequate menstrual products, sanitation and knowledge about proper menstrual hygiene especially in rural areas of developing countries including India.

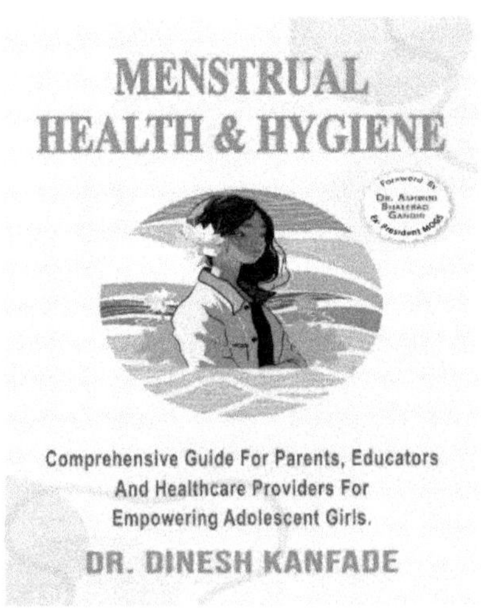